Pregnancy Uncensored

Jocelyn Hayes

BLACK ROSE
writing™

ISBN: 978-1-61296-836-0
PUBLISHED BY BLACK ROSE WRITING
www.blackrosewriting.com

Printed in the United States of America
Suggested retail price $16.95

Pregnancy Uncensored is printed in Adobe Garamond Pro

Melissa Mattey, thank you for being there, for supporting me, stitching me up, and being prepared to fish my poop out of the labor tub. You saw me at my most vulnerable but never made me feel that way. I shall forever be grateful.

Pregnancy Uncensored

Preface

I never intended to write this book. It started out as a few diary entries and ended up as a 50,000-word book detailing my pregnancy journey in all its embarrassing, hilarious, and gory detail. This book is intended to tell you all the things about pregnancy that no one ever told you. I'm breaking down the myth that pregnancy is a magical time and telling it how it really is. No airbrushing. No Instagram filters. It will be gritty. It will be brutal. And you will laugh. But most importantly, for all you ladies out there who are expecting (or trying for, or even just considering kids), I'm telling you that you don't have to fake the "pregnancy glow." You're not alone in feeling that pregnancy is kind of crap.

As you will find out in the course of this book, when I became pregnant I was so certain that I wanted certain things, namely a hospital birth and all the drugs I was legally allowed. But along the way I changed my mind about a lot of things. I ended up doing a home birth with the most wonderful woman I've ever met, my midwife, Melissa Mattey.

Chapter 1– So You Think You Want a Baby?

So there I was, sitting at my desk, aware that I needed to call and make an appointment to have my IUD taken out, procrastinating. I was scared to make the call. After a decade of being on birth control the idea of being without it was terrifying. Since the advent of the pill women have been putting off pregnancy longer and longer. Being pregnant when you're young, to my generation, is seen as a bad thing. We equate it with giving up on our goals and the opportunities feminism has fought so hard to give us.

I'm 27 years old and while intellectually I know that's not that young I don't feel old enough to have children. I mean, I can't even drive for Christ's sake! I don't know how to do a tax return, what dividends means, what the real difference is between political parties, why we're really at war with the middle east, how to organize a mortgage or a pension, what APR stands for, what the difference is between stocks and shares (is there a difference?), how to fix a leaky pipe, when the clocks go back, how to change a fuse, or indeed anything my parents know how to do that I don't.

Don't get me wrong, my parents didn't raise a total dud of a daughter. I do know how to do things like cook, take care of myself, travel safely, and I possess various skills that have landed me several good jobs. But, at 27 years old, I still don't feel like a real adult. I don't feel as grown up as my parents were when they had me, and I think it's a problem common among my generation. We're all still kids. In fact, many people my age STILL live with their parents, and while I know this is often due to us being unable to afford to buy places of our own, having mummy do your laundry and pick up after you long after you're officially an adult isn't helping us grow up any faster. Now, more than ever, it seems socially acceptable to be a teenager well into your thirties.

When I talk to my friends, despite the fact that we'll all soon be approaching 30, they all behave the same as when we were 20. All of my close friends are career focused (and party focused). None of them want children until after the age of 30. None. We're all scared to lose our independence, because you do when you have kids. Your life changes irrevocably. Like Bill Murray says in *Lost in Translation*, "Your life as you know it is gone, never to return."

Of course, children are wonderful, and worth it in the end (so I'm told). But, when confronted with making the phone call to remove my IUD birth control that had been my sperm safety net for the last 5 years, I suddenly wasn't so sure I was ready for my life to change. I was scared. And not just scared about the responsibility of looking after another human being (I know I can do that - I have a husband, after all). I'm scared of being pregnant.

When I was younger I used to get nightmares about being pregnant. Shows like MTV's *Sixteen and pregnant* have terrified my generation and convinced us that getting pregnant when we're young is nothing short of the end of the world. And while I agree that scaring 16 year olds into not getting pregnant is a good idea, there's a fatal flaw in that plan. All my adult female friends are still teenagers at heart! We're in our late twenties and we still have the same reaction to getting pregnant that we did aged 16: "OMG! My life is over. I can't do this. How do I tell my parents?" Yes

I have so many worries about being pregnant. What if having children ruins my body and gives me dreadful stretch marks and slack breasts? Yeah, I'm vain. So what? At least I admit it. What if I get debilitating morning sickness like the Duchess of Cambridge? What if the rollercoaster hormones give me acne? I suffered that for too long as a teenager and an adult that I never want to experience that again. I mean never with a capital "N" and about five billion exclamation marks. What if my child has a disability? I'll be upfront and say I don't want that sort of burden. (Sharp intake of breath as women worldwide label me heartless.) What if I get postpartum depression? I've had a bout of clinical depression before and I never want to re-visit it. What if my child turns out to be a psychopath or a murderer? (Okay, my neuroses may be getting a little out of hand now).

Pick up any baby magazine and you'll see that everyone paints such a glossy, airbrushed picture of pregnancy and motherhood. But I was ten years old when my little brother was born. So I'm not totally ignorant as to what'll be coming my way when I have kids. And let me tell you now, I know it's going to be NOTHING like the adverts on T.V. It won't be anything like what you see on celebrity twitter accounts where supermodels cuddle their newborn lovingly in their blatantly fake "I just woke up like this and everything is fabulous" photos. It's going to be hard. I'll be kissing a good night's sleep goodbye for at least 7 years (more likely 14-15). I'll have to deal with baby vomit on all my clothes, snotty noses, poopy diapers so vile they could knock out a bystander ten feet away, temper tantrums in supermarkets, screaming children that refuse to be placated on planes, and a never-ending list of otherwise "charming" tasks.

Of course, no one tells you about the unpleasant side of children. I only know about it because I experienced some of it firsthand with my little brother. It's like there's some worldwide conspiracy to cover up all the shitty aspects (pardon the pun) of motherhood lest we decide that actually, we'd rather not procreate. We'd rather not deal with five year olds demanding to use the bathroom the moment there's no bathroom in sight despite having been asked twenty times previously if they needed it, or being woken up at 5am by a cascade of wooden toys on your head. We'd rather spend our money on Jimmy Choos, frequently go out to fancy restaurants, sleep in all day on the weekends, go on last minute holidays, keep our sex life active and interesting, and sip on cosmopolitans in our immaculate kitchens whilst wearing vintage Dior. … *Right*.

Perhaps the fact that I actually had a good idea of what I was in for was the reason I was so scared to make that phone call to the clinic. I wasn't sure I was ready to give up the life I had. I wasn't sure I was ready to devote so much of my time to someone that wasn't me or my husband. I know that sounds selfish, but there is a serious element of sacrifice to having children. What you want takes second place over your child's wants and needs, and I wasn't sure I wanted to put myself second. After school, University, and several jobs that I hated, I don't feel I've had much time in my adult life to really do the things that I want to do. I haven't had any real "me" time. And now I hear you asking, "Why are you thinking of getting pregnant if you're not ready?" Well, there are three reasons.

Firstly, my partner is 20 years older than me. Due to his age, I can't afford to wait too long to have children. I knew that when I married him and I chose to marry him anyway. I'd like my children to be able to play with their father before he requires the use of a walking aid.

Secondly, I'm not that young. I'm almost the same age my mother was when she had me. A lot of women these days wait until their thirties, often until their mid-thirties, to have children and then find they have problems conceiving (rates of IVF are higher than ever). Biologically (but not legally) speaking, I've been capable of bearing children for the last 14 years. I'm already getting old in that respect. *Yes*. *yes*.

And thirdly, I don't think anyone is ever truly ready for kids, so now is as good a time as any. If you think you are ready, you're deluded and you have no

9

idea what's about to hit you. <u>No one is ever ready for kids.</u> <u>No one.</u>

I spent a day and a half procrastinating over that phone call. I tidied the house, folded all my clothes (I never fold clothes), did some baking to calm myself down, ran some errands that I'd been putting off forever, and discussed my situation with a select few friends. In the end, I had to reason with myself that if my kids were as cool as my brother eventually turned out to be (yeah, note I said "eventually" there- I disliked him until he was able to talk and he wasn't really "cool" company until he was seven), then it wouldn't be so bad. I picked up the phone and, heart thudding like I was waiting for exam results; I made the appointment to remove my IUD.

Chapter 2- The Vagina Clinic

I hate visiting the vagina clinic (yeah, I know it's got a technical name, but let's just call it what it is). It's about the most awkward experience you can imagine. I decided I hated it immediately upon my first visit to get my IUD put in when they asked to weigh me. I mean, come on! As if it's not already a humiliating enough experience, you want to weigh me with all my clothes on AFTER I've eaten breakfast and drunk about a gallon of coffee? That's NO way to get on a girl's good side.

Next, you have to answer silly questions like, "When was your last period?" (Like I'd know) I've never kept track of the dates of my period. I mean never. I have no idea how long my cycle is and I've only ever known my period was due because I would cry inexplicably for no reason at all in the week it was due and then be outrageously horny the day before it was due. Those were always good enough benchmarks for me, so I never kept track of the dates. But when you're faced with a stern looking nurse, "I don't know" doesn't seem like the appropriate answer.

Finally, when the nurse is done making you feel totally irresponsible for not knowing anything about your monthly cycles, you're asked to strip from the waist down, put your legs in something that resembles a torture contraption with nothing more than a thin sheet of paper to cover your modesty, and wait for the doctor. At this point you usually start to panic about the state of your bikini line, or whether you have any tissue stuck to you down there from the last time you used the bathroom. (Yeah, TMI, I know, but cheap tissue does that - it's a valid concern.)

When the doctor does, at last, arrive, you are faced with one of the weirdest encounters you'll ever have in life. Both of you suddenly turn into small talk experts in an effort to do anything but acknowledge the fact that they're seeing all your bits in more detail than anyone else ever has. Certainly, no man that's ever gone down on me used a glaringly bright lamp and a magnifying glass to do it. But then again, I've not slept with any Sherlock Holmes fanatics.

I feel completely unprepared to be pregnant. I'm not organized enough to work out when I'm ovulating. I don't seem to be capable of taking my vitamins every day, so I'm definitely not going to be taking my temperature every day. I know you're supposed to ovulate 14 days after the start of our period, but based on my period tracking skills, you'd think I'm not capable of counting past the number 5.

Realistically, I reckon I'll have to go for a machine gun approach to getting knocked up and tell the husband that we'll have to bang like crazy for a few months because I can't be bothered to do any mental arithmetic (somehow I don't think he'll have a problem with this).

Furthermore, I have reservations about joining the ranks of pregnant women because there's a whole host of things about them that really irritate me. Like women who announce their baby news by saying, "We're pregnant." WFT is with people who do that? Your husband isn't pregnant. You are! It's either, "I'm pregnant," or, "He got me pregnant." There's no "we" involved in actually being pregnant. That lovely task is left to the women. Because who doesn't want to have to carry a parasite that will take what it needs from your body before you get it for nine months? I'm not kidding here either. If you don't eat enough calcium your unborn baby will force your body to start dissolving your bones so it can have more. Now tell me that's not the behavior of a parasite?

I'm also determined not to be one of those pregnant women that are forever caressing their bump. I don't know why, but it's always annoyed the hell out of me when women constantly do that. Just like I'm not going to be one of those women that creates a Facebook account for their unborn child and makes every social media post baby-to-be related (I've actually de-friended people for this).

"Baby's first croissant today."

"Baby's first taste of tuna today."

"Baby's first hot chocolate today."

UGH! SHUT UP! If I wanted to know what you're eating I'd look at Instagram!

One of the things that bothers me most about children is that women seem to disappear the moment they become a mother. Suddenly, everything you ask them is always linked back to their kids. Now, I don't mind people being proud of their kids and I understand that children are a big part of a mother's life, but when I ask, "How are you?" I really want to know how YOU are doing. Not what little Jimmy got up to yesterday. If it were an English comprehension test, you'd fail for not answering the actual question.

I guess, to summarize, there's a lot I don't like about pregnancy, mothers, and children, and I'm sure I don't even know the half of it yet. I would, in fact, be perfectly happy if someone could drop a five-year-old in my lap so I could skip the baby, toddler and potty training stages altogether and go straight to the school-age stage (yes, I know I could adopt, but my husband doesn't like that idea).

To me, babies are a lot like pet fish, noisy fish. You do everything for them and get very little back. I'm prepared to shock every woman out there by saying, "I don't really like babies." Give me a kid who can talk over a screaming baby any day. Of course, everyone informs me that those sentiments will change when it's my own kid… I guess we'll see.

Chapter 3- Pregnancy Grenade

Folks, we're live. I have now returned from my vagina clinic appointment to have my IUD taken out and not only did the doctor get a good look at my bits, he also got to check my breasts for lumps (they're fine, by the way). I can't help but wonder whether the male doctors are so used to seeing women's bits that they fail to get excited anymore, or whether they're just secret perverts, rating my boobs in their head, "Six out of ten, nice size, not too droopy etc."

As usual, the nurse weighed me and I made the stupid mistake of watching the scale to see what I weigh. So, I got to spend the rest of the day annoyed that the number was higher than I wanted it to be (I was wearing all my clothes and because the appointment was so damn early I hadn't had time for my morning poo! Anyone who weighs themselves seriously knows you don't weigh yourself before you've done your morning bathroom business. That's like adding a whole extra pound right there!), and they took my blood pressure.

"It's a bit high. How are you feeling?"

"Uh, other than the fact that I'm about to strip and no one will be getting pleasure out of it and you're about to pry my innards open with a cold metal speculum and poke around... I'm doing just great, thanks."

This time, unlike my last appointment, I was asked to totally strip and was given one of those backless gowns to wear. Considering the fact that the doctor lifted it up to check out my boobs and abdomen, I had to wonder what the point of the gown was? I mean, he saw everything. I might as well have been naked. Or were we supposed to be keeping my shoulders covered? Because lord knows they're so risqué!

Due to the fact that my choice of birth control over the last 5 years has been a copper IUD that never affected my fertility (unlike hormonal birth control, the copper IUD doesn't stop you ovulating, it just makes the uterus a hostile place for sperm to be, thus preventing pregnancy) the doc warned me that I "could get pregnant very quickly." I felt like adding that at the rate my husband and I do it it's almost a certainty, but I didn't. I was too busy worrying about my bikini line.

I've tried almost every birth control option out there over the years and while IUD's aren't very popular amongst my generation, they're my favorite. I've always had problems with hormonal birth control. The progesterone ones gave me cystic acne and made me cry uncontrollably (and no one wants to shag a spotty, weepy woman) and the estrogen ones made my boobs look like melons (none of my boyfriends complained about this) but they made me gain weight and gave me terrible nausea.

I tried condoms but my boyfriend at the time complained that they cut his enjoyment because he couldn't feel as much, and they kept ripping, meaning I had to keep taking the morning after pill (I don't know what the hell he was doing for that to keep happening- maybe he was sabotaging them?). I even tried a diaphragm but another boyfriend said the spermicidal cream irritated his wang. So that option was out too. All that was left was the copper IUD.

IUD removed, I walked out of the clinic feeling a lot like a grenade that had just had the pin pulled out. Now I feel like a walking, live pregnancy bomb that could go off at any moment. It's a bit scary. My husband was wonderfully supportive, and dare I say it, even a bit mushy about the fact that we're really, seriously trying for kids now and as I tentatively limped out of the clinic with a gait not dissimilar to John Wayne, he got all cuddly and lovey-dovey. It would have been a wonderful, symbolic moment had I not been preoccupied with the fact that the scales had said I weighed 148 pounds instead of 145 when I stood on them.

One good thing about having my IUD out is that my stomach is flatter. I hadn't realized it, but the entire time it was in my lower abdomen was a bit swollen. Now my jeans fit better because the waistband doesn't dig in as much. But I know that joy will be short lived. Soon I'll be in maternity clothes, but from what I hear, maternity jeans are great because you can eat dinner and rather than cutting off the circulation to the lower half of your body your waistband expands with you. (Seriously, fashion people! Why aren't all trousers like that? None of us have a secret desire to be turned into sausages.)

I've got to admit, the moment I went "live" it seemed like the world took notice. I'm not kidding. The first YouTube advert I saw when I got home wasn't some skimpily dressed pop star endorsing some pointless fragrance or diet drink. It was a baby advert! And everywhere I go I notice other women's babies. It's like they're looking at me creepily saying, "You're next." Even in the store I was confronted with a jar of pasta sauce called "Prego." I wanted to scream "Don't rub it in!" at the shelf but that's the behavior of a crazy lady, and I don't want to be known as the woman who shouts at pasta sauce.

My husband and I have sex pretty much every day (yeah, I know I'll be kissing that goodbye too), and the day I had my IUD removed was no exception. However, it wasn't a wonderfully romantic, touching, "We're creating another human being and isn't that amazing?" kind of event. It was more like first time sex. I was shit scared. So much so that it required two shots of rum before I could do it. (Hey, I'm getting my drinking in now before I have to stop.)

I'm genuinely terrified of pregnancy and childbirth. I guess it doesn't help that in my head childbirth looks a lot like that scene in *Alien* where the baby aliens explode out of the humans. Yeah. That definitely doesn't help.

While I was sitting waiting for the doctor at the vagina clinic I had nothing to do but read the information on the walls. There was a poster with a biology textbook style diagram of a pregnant woman with information explaining that happens in each trimester. I was horrified looking at it. I don't want something that huge inside me! <Insert crass joke about "that's what she said"> I don't want my intestines to be up with my lungs! And when I read about what happens to the placenta during the afterbirth, I genuinely wanted to run away and hide in a cupboard. It's lucky they didn't take my blood pressure after I'd read that. I would have broken the machine.

I suppose at some point I'm going to have to start reading pregnancy books. I know there's some stuff I'm not supposed to eat and conflicting advice about whether I'm allowed to workout or not. I guess this part of my life is where my mother will suddenly re-enter my life in a big way. It's normal that teenagers come to the conclusion that their parents know nothing and are totally stupid, and that belief tends to continue until about the age of 23 or 24. Then, when confronted with our first jobs, leases on flats, and often our first serious heartbreaks, our parents suddenly become very wise. And when we have children, they become a God-like font of all knowledge and we end up apologizing profusely for what we put them through. I expect my mother will grow wiser by the day now.

I've had a few days to get used to the idea of really, actually getting pregnant now and I've mostly come to view it as some looming D-day situation. Or should that be B-day? I feel I'm seriously running out of time to do the things I really want to do that will be near impossible to do with children. Once I have a baby, I'll be so shattered that without a coffee addiction more serious than Jordan Belfort's *Wolf of Wall Street* cocaine problem, I'm not going to be able to achieve any of my own goals for a while. But maybe, in a way, that's not such a bad thing. Sometimes we need deadlines to act.

Chapter 4- Parenting Squabbles

A word of advice, don't marry a scientist unless you have the patience of a saint. Normally, I'm a pretty patient person, but sometimes I get annoyed (thus proving I am actually human). Yes, my husband and I have had our first "parenting" argument. It came about because he mentioned he'd read a study about how allowing your baby to sleep with you in bed makes for better, more secure children. (Or something of the sort - to be honest, I stopped listening after the first sentence.) The argument began because I flatly objected. There's no way I want to share my bed with my newborn baby. That may sound heartless, but it's anything but. I'm terrified I'd squash it, or suffocate if it were next to me. I know I wriggle around quite a bit when I sleep and I honestly don't think I could live with myself if I did suffocate my child. Can you imagine the death certificate? "Death by boob."

I know full well that newborn babies can hardly move. It takes them a couple of months to even be able to raise their heads. I remember when my brother was a baby I used to stare at him and wonder how on earth his tiny little neck could hold up his massive head. It was baffling. I don't want to share my bed with something that cannot move away from me if it's being squashed. Of course, being a scientist, my husband then proceeded to tell me I was being irrational and quote statistics of how the chances of me killing my child in my bed were very low.

Okay, let's just pause here for a second. Let me just throw this out there: I've never heard of anyone changing their mind on what they were afraid of because someone quoted statistics to them. I don't care what the statistics are. I'm afraid of it enough that I wouldn't be able to go to sleep, and with enough sleep deprivation, I will turn homicidal and the chances of someone snuffing it in that bed will increase significantly (with the most likely candidate being my husband). And if it happened, I wouldn't be able to cope.

Do you want to know what else I'm irrationally afraid of? Sharks. I've watched every documentary on them I could find, read all the statistics, and I still think that every time I go in the ocean I'm about to become lunch. I cannot go in the ocean alone. Even when I'm with someone, I'm nervous. I hate going past water that's waist deep. Sometimes I even freak out in a swimming pool if I'm alone. (As if there'd ever be a shark in a swimming pool. No, wait, there was in *Thunderball*. My fear is justified.) I find them so scary that I can't even watch a shark documentary with my feet on the floor. Am I being irrational? Yes. Am I likely to ever be bitten by a shark? Not really, no. Do I know that? Yes. Does it change anything? No.

I know a lot of people say we should face our fears, but really, I think that applies to fears that are impacting our everyday lives. Like fear of crowds, or germs. My fears, on the other hand, don't impact my daily life, and are, in fact, TOTALLY AVOIDABLE. Bar some freak sharknado situation, I can't get eaten by a shark if I don't swim in the ocean, and I can't smother my child if they don't sleep with me. That was the argument I made, which to me, sounded perfectly reasonable.

However, accepting my feelings on the matter wasn't a good enough argument for my husband. He needed DATA. It wasn't until he had searched for research and read up on cases of sudden infant death syndrome (SIDS) that he agreed to a compromise and apologized for being pushy. I don't mind the baby being in the same room as me, even in a cot right next to the bed, but I refuse to have it sleep right next to me, or rather, I refuse to sleep next to it. So, scientific journals consulted, we are agreed. The baby gets to sleep right next to the bed, but not in it.

Luckily, we do already agree on many other parenting things. We're both advocates of tough love. I can't stand how parents molly-coddle their children these days. They're terrified of letting them do anything that might result in injury, and what's really sad is that they instill their overbearing fears (of nut allergies, germs, wasp stings, bruises from falling off bikes, risks of climbing trees, pedophiles that could snatch children from the garden, etc.) into their children. Nowadays, children seem to live their paranoid lives wrapped in cotton wool, terrified of anything happening to them (good or bad).

My husband and I currently live in the U.S., and the scaremongering here is off the chart. I could understand parents being wary of letting their children play in the street in say, a big city, but we live in suburbia, where NOTHING happens. The most dangerous thing you will see is someone riding a bicycle without a helmet (and even then, they'll get in trouble for that). It's the safest place I've ever been to in my entire life (and is actually advertised as America's safest city since 2004), and still parents are scared of letting their children play outside. It's utterly absurd.

The schools are just as bad too. One mother (British) forlornly told me that the kids here aren't allowed to run during playtime. They have to walk everywhere. I mean, seriously? WTF?! I understand there's a huge suing culture in the U.S. for accidents, but kids are supposed to run around and lick trees (or whatever). You cannot ban a child from being active and then expect them to sit still in school all day. That's just idiotic beyond belief. If children are actively discouraged from doing exercise, then it's no wonder the U.S. population is slowly heading towards being totally reliant on fatmobiles to get around.

It's really up to the parents to set the tone for how children should react to the inevitable part of childhood that involves bumps, bruises, and an almost guaranteed trip to the hospital. I remember being a nanny to a little girl in London when I was at university. She came running to me one day to show me a bad bruise on her leg. She was clearly expecting me to go, "Oh my God! What did you do? Are you alright?" but instead I just went, "Meh, kids are supposed to be bruised." I spent my youth covered in bumps and scrapes and spent the vast majority of my time looking a lot like I fell through a hedge backwards. Kids do stupid things, and they hurt themselves (usually, not badly). What they learn from that is not to do whatever they were doing again, because, you know… OW! It hurt.

One of the most important discussions we had about children (and one that every couple should have BEFORE you try for children) was what we would do if early testing showed there was something genetically wrong with the baby. My husband asked me what I would want to do and I said, "Abort it. Immediately." I don't expect everyone to agree with me here, but I, personally, don't want to look after a disabled child if I can avoid it. That's just my personal view and you can disagree and call me cruel, but nature is cruel (seriously, sometimes tigers eat their young just because they don't like them). I have the right to choose to abort a healthy fetus for no reason other than I don't want it, so I feel I have equal right to choose to abort a disabled fetus because I don't want it.

It's actually pretty amazing that my husband and I agree on so many things to with children because we've had very different upbringings. He was raised in Canada, by a single mother who worked very hard. He went to state school and was a classic nerd who was bullied a lot. I grew up in England, with two parents. My father worked and my mother was a traditional stay-at-home mother. I went to private school, and then at age 13 I went to boarding school (where bullying was not tolerated so I got to be a bit weird in peace). In comparison to my husband, I had a very privileged upbringing. Add that to the twenty-year age difference and the fact that he's a scientist and I totally suck at math, and you'd think there was no way we could have anything in common. But surprisingly, we get along famously.

Having a sound relationship with your other half is pretty important because children place a MAJOR strain on a relationship. This is another thing no one tells you. Your children are going to do their best to break up your relationship (not intentionally, but they do). The image most people have of children is of how cute they look when they're asleep. Yup, they're cute, but what people don't tell you is that they are the most gifted (and shameless) manipulators you're ever likely to meet. Children learn very quickly EXACTLY where your weak spots are, and they will shamelessly play mummy and daddy off against each other to get what they want.

Picture this: Little girl goes to mummy. "Can I have a sweetie?" she asks. Mummy says no because she'll spoil her dinner. Little girl knows daddy totally has a soft spot for his little princess, so she goes to ask daddy. Daddy says yes. Mummy comes in to find little girl, with candy, sitting on daddy's lap looking at mummy with a smug grin on her face that says, "I totally own daddy and there's nothing you can do about it." Cue huge argument between mummy and daddy.

Or this one: Little boy does something bad. Daddy punishes him by taking away some favorite toy. Little boy goes running to mummy who can't bear to see her golden little boy in tears. Mummy says daddy was just over-reacting and returns said toy. Daddy comes in and is furious that mummy undermined his authority. Mummy gets angry that daddy is "scaring" little boy with his shouting. Cue huge argument between mummy and daddy.

There is a reason the phrases "mummy's boy" and "daddy's girl" exist, and a reason Freud came up with so many theories about children wanting to dispose of one parent and have the other all to themselves. Children want all of your attention and you have to really be on each other's side as parents to not have your children drive a wedge between you. I see it far too often with parents these days. Either they haven't agreed on a parenting style and the conflict of how to discipline their children makes them resent each other (you only have to watch *Nanny 911* to see how much of a problem this is), or they ignore their partner because their child is demanding their attention every second of the day and they give in to it, which also leads to resentment (and dare I say it, the rejection and lack of attention from one's spouse can sometimes lead to an affair).

I don't pretend to be an expert on parenting, but I've had enough of a taste of it, and seen enough of it to know that it's very important to discuss and agree on parenting styles BEFORE you have children. If you can't agree, or continually undermine your partner's authority as a parent, your relationship is going to suffer. And seeing as I'm rather fond of my relationship with my husband, I'm glad we're discussing this all now, because I doubt I'd be able to discuss it reasonably later when I'm cranky, sleep deprived, and full of hormones.

Oh, and I'm just going to share one other piece of wisdom to any prospective mothers. When my Mother was pregnant with my brother she told me I wouldn't have to change diapers. It was a huge lie. A bigger lie even than Santa. I'm not going to be fooled again. My husband told me, "You won't have to change all the diapers. I'll do my fair share." This time I'm not going to let that slide. I'm going to make him sign and date that statement and I'm going to frame it and hang it over the nappy changing table so he can't deny it. I highly recommend you do the same.

Chapter 5- I'm Pregnant

The vagina clinic doctor wasn't wrong. I did get pregnant very quickly, very quickly indeed. By my husband's calculations (we're using his because my math sucks) I got pregnant the day or the day after my IUD was taken out, because lo and behold, two weeks later I found myself staring at that little white and pink stick watching a second blue line appear in the box.

I've taken my fair share of pregnancy tests over the last eight or so years, not because I was irresponsible about birth control, but because I was paranoid that I'd be in that 1% for whom it wasn't effective, but I've never seen that second blue line appear. My first reaction was to smile, and then I started to feel overwhelmed. Not with joy, but with worry, and a certain degree of annoyance, because now I really do have to stop drinking. I don't drink much, but I have so few vices that missing that one glass of red wine in the evening was a depressing concept.

If I'm honest, I knew I was pregnant before I took the test. In fact, it was what prompted me to go buy one in the first place. There had been several indications, my period was late (but so had the previous one been, so I didn't take that as a given sign), I had been feeling a lot more tired than usual, and I had occasionally felt quite sick when eating. But none of those were strong enough signs for me to do anything. My period has often kept to a fashionably late schedule, I've suffered on and off with anemia for a decade, so tiredness is nothing unusual, and I have Celiac Disease, meaning I often feel unwell when I eat if there's some sneaky ingredients in my food that I'm not supposed to have. No. The one thing that forced me out to the pharmacy was my boobs.

The last time I tried going on the pill it lasted for all of eleven days. I hated it because in those eleven days my boobs inflated like watermelons. Not only was it painful, I psychologically hated it. Usually, when your body changes you have a chance to get used to it because the change is gradual. You don't grow two feet overnight, nor do you put on twenty pounds overnight. With the pill, however, I felt as though I'd woken up with a boob job. It felt like someone had suddenly stuck two ginormous foreign objects on my chest. They didn't feel a part of me and it was quite distressing. Needless to say, I was mega relieved when I came off the pill and my boobs went back to normal.

The day I made my trip to buy a pregnancy test it was because my boobs felt the same as they did on the pill. BAM! Overnight, I woke up with pumped up hooters. I'm aware that that sounds like a boy's wet dream, and even some girls' dream come true, but for me it was more of a nightmare, not least because I now didn't fit into my very new, beautiful, expensive bras and no, I will not wear bras that don't fit. The four-boob look is NEVER in season. NEVER.

I had contemplated taking the pregnancy test in the store so I could find out immediately if my suspicions were correct, but there's just not enough privacy in American bathrooms. They have some weird obsession with making the doors as see-through as physically possible. In England, bathroom doors generally go from ceiling to floor with no gap underneath the door and certainly no gap between the door and the frame. Here, in the U.S., the doors are only about five-foot-high, have a gap under the door so large that a child can crawl under to see what you're up to, and have cracks either side of the door frame so big that anyone who cared to look could see you. It's an invasion of privacy that I simply cannot get used to (sometimes I get stage fright and have to put my fingers in my ears and close my eyes so I can pretend I'm alone in order to pee), and not an environment in which I want to find out the course of my future, so I took the test home.

I didn't tell my husband that I suspected I was pregnant, nor did I tell him that I was going to take a pregnancy test. I just took it in silence, watched with a mixture of happiness and horror as the second blue line appeared, and went to find him for a hug. He was working, as usual. I sat down on his lap and placed the pregnancy test on the desk. He actually didn't notice it at all until I pointed at it. Then he laughed and said, "I thought you looked more worried than usual." (As a side note: I do find it a bit strange that you announce life changing news by putting your urine in front of someone. I can't think of any other situation where you'd give someone a stick of your pee and say, "You can celebrate now." If that happened anywhere else in life you'd report that person to the mental health authorities.)

My husband is normally a fairly emotional person, and in other circumstances I would have placed good money on the probability of him crying at such news. However, he was married before me, and they tried for kids for several years. He had heard this news quite a few times before with no success (unfortunately, none of the pregnancies worked out). So instead of him breaking down with joy, he just smiled and said, "I think we should make really sure you're pregnant." Yes, you read that correctly. Instead of the Disney scenario where the man gets all emotional and tells the woman how much he loves her and they cry and get giddy and excited, my husband wanted to shag, again, just to be extra sure I really was knocked up.

This has actually been a bit of a downside of being with someone substantially older than me. There are things that should be momentous occasions in my life, but he's done them before, so isn't that excited about them. I do want to clarify that I'm not a princess who wants to celebrate over every tiny thing, but my tolerance levels only go so low. Let me give you an example of where I draw the line. Our wedding day was in the middle of three weeks of dog sitting for one of my husband's colleagues (I wasn't thrilled about it but he wanted to gatecrash their big house for a while instead of our flat). However, one of the dogs was not house-trained, which we were only told about when we picked up the keys. (Dog owners: if you do this, you should be ashamed! Never inflict your untrained pet on someone without fair warning!) This meant that on my wedding day, instead of having a romantic evening with my husband, I was cleaning up dog shit from the bathroom mat (I now detest Chihuahuas – handbag rodents). It was not what I had had in mind for my first night of supposed marital bliss.

I'm the first person among my close friends to get pregnant and I have conflicting feelings about it. Unlike most women, I'm not over the moon and in a strange way, I feel a bit emotionless about it. I'm not desperate to have children. I think I'd make a good mother, but I am not baby gaga. I'm probably going to rob my female friends of a chance to go baby nuts. I don't want a baby shower, I don't want to talk endlessly about babies, I don't want gifts of new baby things (they'll either throw up on it or outgrow it quickly anyway- we'll get second hand stuff), and I don't want them to think I'm precious or fragile. I'm a strong, capable woman and I don't mean that in the figurative sense. I'm physically strong. The day after I told my husband I was pregnant he said, "I guess you're not supposed to lift anything heavy now." I immediately replied, "What?! I was doing push-ups yesterday!"

Bar the exhaustion of being pregnant limiting my activity, I don't intend to stop working out. There's a lot of bad press about women exercising while pregnant, and to be frank, I'm not sure where it comes from. Women respond to pregnant women in the gym the same way they respond to pregnant women asking for a glass of wine: with horror. This cushy existence of ours where we sit on the couch all day binge watching Netflix with a box of chocolates is a new thing. I'm not saying I'm going to suddenly attempt a deadlift record while pregnant, but I sure as hell won't be sitting on my butt pretending I'm made of glass for the entire pregnancy. Our ancestors did lots of exercise while pregnant in the search for food, and I intend to maintain my exercise as much as I can too.

Chapter 6– Pregnancy "Diet"

While we're on the subject of food, I take massive issue with the way most pregnant women approach food. The way I see it, they just use it as an excuse to get fat. I see it everywhere. Pregnant women sit with an entire cheesecake in front of them and when you dare to suggest they don't need to eat the entire thing they indignantly reply, "I'm eating for two!" But, surely we need a sanity check here? If you think you're eating for two, you're deluded. You're using that as your defense to eat whatever you want with absolutely no consideration for the calorie content.

Firstly, you are NOT eating for two fully grown adults. At the start, you are eating for you and something the size of a TADPOLE! It's well documented that women actually ONLY need to eat about 250-300 calories more when pregnant. That's one snickers bar. Yup. One. Not an entire cake or a two-liter vat of chocapocalypse ice cream. Secondly, what nutritional value does cake or ice cream have? Seriously? Practically none. Sugar is not a nutrient. If you're really worried about your baby getting enough food, you should be trying to eat more vegetables, lean meats, good fats, and complex starches. Pregnancy is NOT a glorified excuse to go on a nine-month binge of biblical proportions.

One of the reasons baby weight is so hard to lose is because women are deluding themselves with the notion that because they are pregnant they can eat whatever they want. A generation or two ago it was almost unheard of for women to gain more than twenty pounds of baby weight. Yet today, women are frequently gaining over fifty pounds! What on earth are they doing? Having ice cream administered intravenously?

I already have a restricted diet due to health reasons (I have autoimmune problems and have altered my diet accordingly). I don't eat any grains or beans (none at all- coffee is a bean and so is chocolate). I don't eat any dairy. I don't eat sugar. I don't eat potatoes (they're a nightshade and I can't tolerate them). I don't eat eggs or nuts, and I don't eat anything with artificial colors, sweeteners or additives.

Of course, the first reaction people have when I tell them about my diet is, "Oh my God. You must be deficient. Where do you get your vitamins?" The answer is you can get all the vitamins you need for a fairly limited range of foods: good quality meats, fish, dark green vegetables, broccoli, etc. In fact, for those of you that don't believe me, here's a list I put together to reassure my Mother. If it's good enough to stop my Mother from panicking (and she's one of those people that thinks milk is high in calcium because it's white- Mum, it's white because it's an emulsion of fat and water, not because it's liquid calcium), it ought to be good enough to reassure you too (but do check with a professional before altering your diet. I am not a qualified dietician. This is just what I do):

Vitamin A: Cod-liver oil, carrots, leafy vegetables,

Vitamin B1 (Thiamine): Fish, pork, squash, vegetables

Iodine: Iodized salt, some seafood, kelp, and seaweed

Iron: Leafy green vegetables, shellfish (not when you're pregnant), red meat, liver

Magnesium: Leafy green vegetables, halibut, avocados, bananas, kiwi fruit, and shrimp

Manganese: Fish, spinach, kale

Molybdenum: Leafy green vegetables

Phosphorus: Beef, chicken, halibut, salmon

Potassium: Broccoli, leafy green vegetables, bananas

Selenium: Organ meats (like liver), salmon, halibut

Zinc: Red meat

Vitamin B2 (Riboflavin): Dark meat chicken, and cooked beef

Vitamin B3 (Niacin): Poultry, fish, meat

Vitamin B6: Bananas, light-meat: chicken and turkey, spinach

Vitamin B12: Beef, salmon, poultry

Vitamin C (Ascorbic Acid): Citrus fruits, red berries, broccoli, cauliflower, sprouts, spinach

Vitamin D: Salmon; and sunlight

Vitamin E: Leafy green vegetables

Folate (Folic Acid): Dark leafy vegetables

Vitamin K: Leafy green vegetables like parsley, chard, and kale, broccoli

Calcium: Broccoli, dark leafy greens like spinach and rhubarb,

Chromium: Beef, turkey, fish, broccoli
Copper: Organ meats (like liver), seafood

Notice how often meat, fish and dark green vegetables came up? Do I need grains to be "healthy"? No I don't.

I understand that pregnant women get cravings and they sit on their butts because they're tired and worried something might happen to the baby if they do anything too strenuous, but I refuse to buy into the notion that it's okay to do NOTHING at all and to eat whatever you want because "that's what's good for the baby." That's bullshit.

If women are so worried about what's good for the baby they'd question whether it's wise to eat their weight in candy when pregnant. You wouldn't let a three-year-old gorge themselves on sugar. So why is appropriate for you to do it while pregnant? You're effectively doing the same thing; giving your child a massive sugar rush. Unless you want your baby training for the Olympic gymnastics team inside your womb, you really should lay off the sugar. Similarly, with exercise, there are plenty of exercises specifically designed for pregnant women, yoga, ballet, swimming etc. Unless you're too sick or too big to move, there's really no excuse. At the risk of upsetting a lot of women: pregnancy is not an excuse to be a lazy, fat slob.

Chapter 7- Baby Announcements And Miscarriage Taboos

There is a lot of dispute about when you should tell people you're pregnant. Commonly, people wait until after the first three months because that's the period when you're most likely to miscarry. I agree that it's probably unwise to broadcast a pregnancy to the entire world until a little way down the line, but I see nothing wrong with telling your nearest and dearest straight away, and that's exactly what I did. Want to know what they said? "Congratulations, but you might still miscarry. So be careful."

WTF?! I'm not joking. Everyone I told first said congratulations, and then immediately warned me I might miscarry. How on earth is that an appropriate response? Firstly, I'm AWARE I might miscarry. I don't need to be reminded by every person I tell (after the third or fourth warning it gets depressing). Secondly, why is it okay to taint good news with a foreboding warning? You would never say, "Congratulations on the engagement but he might still cheat on you." Nor would you ever say, "Congratulations on the new job but they might still fire you." So why is it appropriate to say, "Congratulations on your pregnancy but you might still miscarry"?

I know that miscarriages are a bit of a taboo subject but I don't see why women are expected to keep the news of early pregnancy to themselves. Surely, they should be allowed to tell their best friends, family, and boss that they're pregnant because if they do miscarry they'll need their support and maybe some time off work. Why is it that in the 21st century we are still treating miscarriages like some dirty, dark secret? They're not unusual, nor should they be shameful. This notion that I'm not supposed to tell anyone I'm pregnant "in case I miscarry" is, to me, very antiquated.

I've been warned by friends about how devastated some of their friends were when they miscarried but (unpopular opinion warning) I don't think I would be THAT devastated if I do miscarry. I'm not a particularly emotional person when it comes to baby stuff and I should say that I'm also pro-abortion (no) I've never had one but I believe in my right to have one if I so wish).

At this point, as far as I'm concerned, I'm not really carrying "a baby." I'm carrying a collection of cells the size of a sesame seed. It's not a person yet and if my body aborts it, then I expect it did so for good reason, because there was something wrong with the fetus. And given that I don't want to look after a disabled child if I can avoid it, I doubt I'd get very upset about a miscarriage. I'm far more likely to view it as a narrow escape from a lifelong burden I don't want. (FYI - I'm aware that my views would be considered by many people as controversial, and maybe even heartless, but they're just my opinions. You don't have to agree with me.)

It's funny, but the only person who doesn't seem to be freaking out about my pregnancy is me. My friends and family have asked me if I'm taking it easy, whether it's safe for me to fly over and visit at Christmas, whether it's safe for me to go through the body scanner at LAX, whether I should upgrade to business class (I'm not fat yet!), whether I'm getting enough folic acid in my diet… blah, blah, blah. Thankfully, on my last Skype call with my parent's dad did cut mum's fretting short by reminding her that humans have been having babies for thousands of years without all this fuss.

Initially, I told my parents I was two weeks pregnant but I've since found out my math was incorrect (what a surprise!). Apparently, they calculate your due date from the first day of your last period, rather than from the day you got pregnant. So, when you do get pregnant, you're already considered two weeks pregnant. (To be frank, it sounds like someone with my math skills came up with this system). So, I'm now five weeks pregnant, not three weeks pregnant, and when I found this out I felt like someone had stolen two weeks of my life. I'm two weeks closer to giving birth than I thought I was. Had my husband not been in the room at the time I would have been shouting, "Give it back you time stealing internet machine!" at the online due date calculator.

However, due to this black hole of lost time, it does now mean that I should be in England when I'm eligible for my first ultrasound scan. I'm actually relieved about that, because I know how the UK health system works. I have a major issue with the health system in the U.S. and if we didn't have to be here for my husband's work, I would not choose to be pregnant here. In fact, I've already told my husband point blank that if I get seriously ill he's to put me on the first plane back to the UK. Long term illnesses in the U.S. are expensive affairs and I'd rather be ill in a country that won't try and take my house from me due to extortionate medical bills (I'm a dual national - I have the right to healthcare system of a country I'm a citizen of).

When I was looking at the due date webpage it gave me a calendar with milestones and pictures. I had several problems with it. Firstly, Yuk! The pictures were gross! They looked like something out of a bad science fiction film. I wish I could have unseen them. Now I feel like I have some mutant blob-creature growing inside me. Secondly, some of the information seemed pointless. Like informing me when the baby can see light. Uh... am I missing something here? Last I checked my womb didn't come with a disco ball and strobe lighting. Why do I need to know when it can see light? I'm not phosphorescent. It's pitch bloody black in there!

I'm sort of getting the feeling that I'm not going to be one of those women that's "at their peak" when pregnant. I'm mostly at my peak with a glass of wine in my hand (my second glass, truth be told). I am dreading certain aspects of being pregnant, like antenatal classes. Do I have to do those? You know the ones I mean; the ones where you sit there with your partner and practice breathing hard for when you give birth. I don't want to do that. I'm not sure whether I'd want to collapse into a fit of giggles or die of embarrassment. Besides, who's to say I won't have a C section?

My Mother had a C section for all her children, and due to babies getting bigger and bigger in general, they seem to be getting more common. While I feel being cut open wouldn't be a particularly pleasant experience, I reckon it might actually be preferable to giving birth. I loathe the current notion in the media that if you have a C section you're "too posh to push." To hell with that! Posh or not, I'd rather not ruin my vagina by pushing something that big out of my nether regions. I happen to quite like my nether regions just as they are and to borrow a phrase from the comedian Sarah Millican, "I quite like my downstairs as it is. I'm certainly not looking to get an extension."

It's still a bit early to be making any decisions, but we have considered whether it'd be worth me flying back to the UK to give birth. I'm considering it for two reasons: free healthcare, and that's where my parents are. I'm aware that me giving birth isn't all about me. It's about my family too. My sister will become an Aunt, my brother will become and Uncle (at 17 years old, I guess he'll be the "cool" Uncle), and my parents will become grandparents. Seeing as my father can't fly to the U.S. for medical reasons (the travel insurance would be outrageous and if he had to go to hospital, the bill would be silly) then it makes sense for me to consider giving birth in the UK so they can all be involved. The only drawback is that we'd have to fly back to the U.S. with a baby.

I am generally against babies on flights. Certainly, my parents didn't take my brother on any long-haul flights until he was at least five years old. Taking babies on long flights is not only upsetting to passengers, it's upsetting for the parents of the baby too. Babies don't give a shit how loud they scream (and trust me, in that tin can it's deafening), but the parents do. And to make matters worse, passengers give parents a really hard time about not being able to shut their baby up.

I honestly don't know why airlines don't do family friendly flights and adult only flights. They should. Cinemas and restaurants do it. The people without children would be happier (because they can sip their gin and tonic in peace) and the people with children would be happier (because they wouldn't be getting death stares from all the passengers that don't have children.)

My dad always said you can tell who has children and who doesn't because when your child is in the throes of a tantrum the people who have kids smile at you sympathetically and the people who don't have kids throw you disgusted looks that say, "Why can't you control your child?" However, in a supermarket, you can just walk out. On a plane… you're stuck. Beyond gagging your child, there's not much you can do to reduce the noise levels of a screaming baby. And seeing as I'm not rich enough to charter a private plane, I'm likely to have to join the ranks of embarrassed first time parents that want to die and disappear into a hole because their baby won't shut up on the plane. I don't think my husband would care (he doesn't care what anyone thinks, to the extent that he wears his socks upside down) but I would feel awful.

Finding ways to make parents of small children feel bad almost seems to be a sport, where anyone can have a go. There is always someone out there ready to tell you what you're doing wrong (and quite often, it's people that don't have kids). I'm already bracing myself for the inevitable tsunami of unwanted advice that will come my way when I become a Mother. However, I have decided to create some filters. I will always accept advice given WHEN I ASKED FOR IT! I will consider unwarranted advice from people who have kids, and I will ignore advice from people that have never had kids and have no experience with children whatsoever, and advice from people who have badly trained pets. If you can't train your dog not to shit on the carpet, then no way am I listening to your advice on parenting.

Chapter 8– Sobbing Over Bras and Trouble Making Friends

I have never really liked my body that much but at least in the year before I got pregnant I'd finally come to a point where I didn't hate it. I had a lot of problems with my body as a teenager and young adult, many of which still linger with me today. I was the first in my class at school to get a bra and I'll never forget how one girl came up behind me and pinged the strap before running to tell the whole class. She made me feel awful and I never really forgave her for it.

My boobs grew very quickly. At the age of 13 I was wearing a B cup and by the time I was 16 I wore an E cup. A 36 E (which is pretty darn big - think Christina Hendricks big). I hated my boobs. I hated the ugly purple stretch marks I had gotten from them growing so big so fast, I hated boys' fascination with them, I hated how I couldn't find a single sports bra that really eliminated "bounce" and I hated that no pretty little tops fit me. I also weighed quite a bit more than I do now, which didn't help. I was never truly "fat" but in my eyes I was a whale.

One of the big problems I had in my teenage years was undiagnosed anemia. I developed a reliance on sweets, coffee, and white toast to help get me through the crippling exhaustion I felt, but of course, with sugar comes weight gain. This, in turn, resulted in some pretty extreme body hating on my part. I tried a load of stupid faddy diets. I exercised like a maniac, despite the anemia, and I began to abuse laxative pills. Ironically though, none of those resulted in weight loss (just a lot of time reading on the toilet).

As I neared the age of 25 I lost about two stone and my weight dropped to around 145 pounds and for the first time since I was about 14 I didn't hate what I saw in the mirror. Sure, I wasn't perfect and had I had the powers of an airbrush I would have gone to town on myself like a Vogue cover, but at least my reflection didn't (in my eyes) look like a hippo in a dress anymore. I knew I didn't have washboard abs and my boobs weren't as perky as I would have liked them to be, but I had finally come to terms with what I saw in the mirror, and decided I was okay.

Now, of course, that's all out of the window. Just when I'd decided I was okay with the way I looked, everything started to change. Today was a momentous day. Due to my newly inflated boobs, I had to dig out my old bras from when I was fatter and put away my nice, new ones. I actually cried. I know that sounds pathetic, but it is quite distressing watching your body rapidly change in ways you don't want it to. I just wanted to collapse into my underwear drawer and scream, "I WANT MY SMALLER BOOBS BACK!"

The other day I was reading an article about Lara Stone, the Dutch supermodel, who was talking about how hard she found it to deal with the way her body changed when she was pregnant and how alarming she found the whole experience. Now, I know she's a supermodel so she has the right to worry because her body is her meal ticket, but it was the first time I had heard any "celebrity" say anything less than glowing about pregnancy.

No one really talks about how hard it is to emotionally deal with changes to your body, and certainly no one goes so far as to discuss the fact that they resent their baby for ruining their body. To say such a thing would be considered blasphemy! But here I am, saying loud and clear, I am pissed off that my baby to be has turned my boobs into an anime fantasy! Not only do they feel absurdly huge, they're painful too. It hurts when my husband hugs me tightly and it hurts when I lie on my stomach, which is the only way I fall asleep. I am going to be so screwed when my stomach gets too big for me to sleep on my stomach. Maybe we'll just have to cut a hole in the mattress so I can let it all hang down.

I'm also scared that these changes to my body will make me subject to the common game on public transport of "fat or pregnant?" In a way, I do feel sorry for men. They're supposed to give up their seats to pregnant women, but there are so many fat women now that it's hard to know who's who, and lord help you if you get it wrong. Women slay men so badly these days for offering them seats and holding doors open that they've mostly stopped trying. I love having the door held open for me. I know I can do it myself, but most men are genetically stronger than me, so why not let them hold it open for me? It's polite and it makes me feel like a lady. I'd hold the door open for them if I got there first too. I'm sick of "feminism" dictating that no one is allowed to help me.

I had another teary moment when I started packing up some of my clothes for when we move house in the New Year. I figured I'd just go through my wardrobe and store anything that I won't be able to wear until my boobs deflate and my stomach becomes flat(ish) again. I ended up packing away three quarters of my clothes. They're just clothes (and my husband is barely containing his glee at my newly enhanced rack), but to me it was upsetting putting all those clothes away. It was like putting part of my life in a box, a part that I might not see again. Once I become a mother, I might not get to wear those little party dresses again, certainly not in suburbia. Not unless I want to become known as "the slutty mom" who picks her kid up from daycare in a dress so tight you can see what she had for breakfast.

I am slightly worried about making friends here in the U.S. because I have always found it very difficult to make female friends as an adult. Most of my female friends are back in England, and I made them when I still thought it was fashionable to wear Lion King leggings. They were friendships forged in my ugly duckling days, where we weren't competing for men, and in fact, fancying the same guy wasn't a problem. It merely meant you could talk about them endlessly without anyone getting bored.

My solution to the adult friend making dilemma was to mostly have male friends (or gay friends) because they were easier to get close to and that way I didn't have to deal with female jealousies. And that worked just fine, until my male friends got girlfriends. You see, I'm a fairly attractive woman. Don't get me wrong. I'm no supermodel, but I've never had any problem getting attention from men, and that's become a bit of a problem when it comes to making friends. Women don't like to have friends that are prettier than they are. Yes. I said it. All you feminists can go mental at me now. I bashed my own sex. But it's true. You only need to look at the internet to see how cruel people are to people who are better looking than they are.

Women who don't know me pretty much seem to hate me on sight because they think I'll steal their man. And that attitude goes the same for my male friends' girlfriends. They think I'll steal their boyfriend and more often than not, they either ban my friends from seeing me or insist on being present at all times. Making friends as an adult is a much more complicated process than when you're a kid because the issue of attraction is there, and making friends as an attractive woman is even more difficult.

I've never had a big group of female friends either. For the most part, I find women too annoying. In particular, I don't like how they don't fight fair. My few female friends are like me: direct, to the point, and not overly-emotional about silly stuff. I don't have the patience to listen to women regale me with self-inflicted dramas. Maybe I'm being overly cruel in generalizing women as unfair, gossipy, drama queens, but it's hard not to when these are some of the actual conversations I've had with "friends":

Female 1: "He never does anything around the house. I do everything!"
Me: "Did you ever ask him to do stuff?"
Female 1: "No. I shouldn't have to. He should just know."
Me: "Uh. Men are stupid. You have to ask. If you don't ask, you don't have the right to be angry they didn't do something you didn't ask them to do because they couldn't read your mind."
Female 1: "No. I want him to offer. I don't want to ask."
Me: <Facepalm>

Female 2: "I'm so angry with my boyfriend."
Me: "Why?"
Female 2: "He went out drinking until 3am last night!"
Me: "Did you tell him it was okay to go?"
Female 2: "Yes, but it wasn't."
Me: "But you didn't tell him that?"
Female 2: "No. He should have guessed it. It was obvious!"
Me: <Facepalm>

Female 3: "I bought my boyfriend a really nice birthday present."
Me: "Uh, can you actually afford that?"
Female 3: "No."
Me: "Then take it back. Get something less expensive. He won't care."
Female 3: "No."
Me: "Why not? You seriously can't afford that."
Female 3: "I know. But if he messes up in our relationship again I get to go, 'Look at what I got for you, even when I couldn't afford it. I put myself in debt for you and this is how you treat me?'"
Me: "That's messed up."

You get the idea.

I'm sure I will meet people through my kids, but I'm not really sure it'll make making friends any easier. It's hard to make friends with couples. Couples seem to have their guard up more than single people. I often feel you don't really get to know the individuals very well. My husband didn't believe me when I said that, but I asked him, "How many of your friends knew what your relationship with your ex was really like?" He replied that practically none of them were aware of the problems they had because they hid it really well. And that's exactly my point. Couples almost seem to have a PR agent run over things before any information comes to light. Everything always has to be presented as if it's The Lego Movie- everything is Awesome!

However, I don't want friends that only give me an edited version of events because that'll make me feel shit about how imperfect my life is. I want real friends that I can trust, friends who won't go gossiping about me to other women because my life isn't airbrushed. I want friends that when I call them and say, "I've had a shit day. Baby Jane drew on all the walls with my lipstick and I've spent three hours cleaning them. Please come over with emergency wine," they'll not bat an eyelid. My old friends in London would do that. I'm not sure I'll find that here, not when everyone is so guarded and worried about public opinion.

My husband and I have discussed whether we'll stay here in the U.S. permanently and the answer is likely, no. Neither of us is particularly keen for our kids to turn out like your typical suburban American teenager. Take this as an example. The other day, my husband overheard this conversation in the hot tub:

Female 1: "OMG! The other day I was somewhere where all the houses looked different!"
Female 2: "Yeah, that's from before they had urban planning."
Female 1: "Wow!"

I honestly don't think I will be able to take it if my kids sound like they've nothing but cotton wool between their ears, but in many ways, I can't blame the kids here. In suburban America children are exposed to so few cultural experiences that I can't really blame them for being shallow and vacuous. It's not their fault. There's literally nothing to do but sunbathe, shop, and eat. All I can do is do my best to prevent my kids from turning out like that. I am hoping to move back to the UK (to London) in the next ten years. Sooner, if we can afford it. The U.S. is great for many reasons, but suburbia is not renowned for churning out the most capable, open-minded, and world-wise kids.

Chapter 9- Fatigue and The Caffeine Wasteland

The word "fatigue" doesn't quite seem to cover the extent of the exhaustion I feel. I feel like I've been steamrollered by a bus. And do you know the worst part of it? I can't have more tea or coffee to make it easier to bear, because yup. You guessed it. I'm not allowed much caffeine due to the micro blob growing inside me. If I didn't already resent it for what it's done to my boobs, I'd certainly resent it now.

I haven't been severely anemic for years, but I once was, and this is exactly what it felt like. I was so tired that all I ever wanted to do was lie down. I used to find it so exhausting walking back to my boarding house after school that the only way I could keep going was to keep telling myself, "Just put one foot in front of the other. One step at a time." And when I did get back to my room, I'd plonk my books on my desk, flop on the bed and (I am not exaggerating here) not move for a solid twenty minutes.

I honestly could not be happier that I don't work in an office anymore. There is no way I'd be able to be pregnant at work or indeed hide the fact that I'm pregnant (if you're going by the "don't tell anyone until the first three months are over in case you miscarry" thing). The only time I've felt this bad at work before was when I was on heavy medication for tonsillitis and I was so tired I almost fell asleep sitting on the countertop with my head against the kitchen cupboard as I waited for the kettle to boil.

NO ONE WARNED ME ABOUT THIS! No one told me I'd turn into a complete zombie for the first three months! I'm so pathetic that in the morning all I can do is listlessly raise my arm towards my water as if I'm on my death bed, and I find stairs so exhausting that my husband has to push me up them (not that he minds- he gets to grab my butt in front of people).

If everyone feels like this then how is it okay for employers to expect you to work a full day and be just as productive as before you were pregnant? Sure, you get maternity leave after you have a baby, but what about when your body's busy making one?! The last time I felt this tired my iron levels were so low that I almost qualified for a blood transfusion! And while that was pretty serious, it did give me the somewhat interesting side effect of being so pale that my skin glowed in bright sunlight, which was pretty cool. Forget sparkly Twilight vampires. I freaking glowed!

Thankfully, I have a wonderful husband, who is being very sympathetic (or perhaps I just look so pathetic that it's warranted- who knows?). I googled pregnancy fatigue and I was genuinely sad about many of the posts I read on various forums. There were many women online complaining that their partner thinks they're just hamming it up and using fatigue as an excuse to stay in bed and not do anything. The most I can manage in a day is to tidy the house and maybe walk to the shops, and that's with several lie downs in between.

Companies almost go out of their way to make being pregnant a nightmare (what with you not being able to ask about maternity benefits in interviews or you'll ruin your chances, and your colleagues calling you a slacker when you're off sick for exhaustion or morning sickness), we sure don't need our partners joining in on the "let's call the pregnant women a liar" game.

I'm sure that there probably exist some women who do milk the pregnancy thing for all it's worth so they can be treated like a princess, but that's not most women. Most of us, I'll bet, would do anything to feel normal again, and if there was a way to magically delegate baby making into, say, a chicken egg that we only have to sit on, we'd do it in a heartbeat. I'd happily sit on an egg for nine months if it meant I didn't have to feel this exhausted all the time. Mind you, being a clever species I'm sure we'd invent some sort of incubator to literally babysit for us.

I'm no stranger to exhaustion, but I am a stranger to having all my tools in the anti-fatigue toolbox removed. This time around, I don't have my trusty mochas and peanutty goodness chocolate bars to rely on (having given both those things up due to my autoimmune issues). But even if I was still able to eat those, I can't have too much of them anyway. Too much caffeine is bad for the baby and too much sugar just gives me restless leg syndrome at night (which is so frustrating you just end up wanting to chop your legs off). In short, I have no pick-me-ups to well, pick me up when I feel like a sad two-day old helium balloon that's pathetically limping along at waist height.

Of course, there are plenty of healthy foods out there, but they don't pack much of a punch with fatigue this extreme. When my husband hands me a banana I feel a bit like a picture I once saw of the cookie monster surrounded by fruit saying, "What the hell is this crap?" I like bananas, but they don't seem to put even a small dent in the overwhelming surge of sleepiness I'm snowed in under, though my husband takes considerable pleasure in feeding me one in the morning. Men! They never grow up.

Something I have been very careful about is to try not to start a game of "I'm more tired than you" with my husband. That's dangerous territory when you get into it, because you're no longer a team. You're now competitors. In fact, just the other day I read an article in The Daily Mail (yes, I like my news a little sensationalized- sue me) about a study on three couples where the aim was to see who really was more tired, the mum or the dad. In two out of the three cases, it turned out the dad was more tired (though neither gloated about it lest they invite their wife's wrath). But what really struck me in the article was how resentful each parent had become of the other.

I understand that sleep, like silence, and time to oneself, is a precious commodity as a parent, but there's no reason for a relationship to turn sour over it. I've always hated people who play the "I have it worse than you game." Not only do they do their level best to belittle your feelings, I feel they often actively make their own lives harder than they need to be to make sure they win that game.

Me: "I'm quite tired because work has been stressing me out."
Friend 1: "Well at least you don't have to do your boss's work as well as your own and half the people on your team's!
Me: "Lodge a complaint or quit if it's that bad. Don't put up with and complain about absurd circumstances and do nothing about them just so you can play the martyr game."

I suppose the most depressing thing about being this tired is that it's somewhat killed my sex life. I say "somewhat" because we're still having sex at least every two days, but I'm so tired that I've only had one orgasm in the last 5-6 weeks. For the most part, I just lie there like a starfish and do my best to at least join in a bit.

Sex during pregnancy and sex when you have a newborn is a very touchy subject. I get the impression that a lot of women feel it's a duty they should be "let off." I have two issues with that sentiment. First, if you feel sex with you partner is a chore, that's very sad. Second, by thinking you should be allowed to forgo sex, you're overlooking how important sex is in a relationship. When you think about it, sex is the glue that binds couples together. It's a special something that you only have with your partner. Remove that and your relationship is no different from the relationship you have with friends you love.

Furthermore, it's not really that hard to lie there with your legs open. Seriously, I don't buy the excuse, "I'm too tired for sex." What you really mean is, "I'm too tired for me to orgasm, so we're not having sex." Now, that may be fine for a while (depending on your partner's sex drive) but you're going to reach a point where you're neglecting your partner's needs. <Cue feminist outrage>

Look, I'll be brutally honest. Sex is a biological need, just like food and sleep, and you cannot deny your partner it for long without consequences. My husband has a very high drive, and yes, I get tired too sometimes. But I don't often say "no" to him. What I do sometimes say is, "I'm pretty shattered so don't wait for me. It's not gonna happen. Just go for gold." Spreading my legs for ten minutes every other day is hardly that demanding, and often, I do enjoy it a bit once we get going, even if I don't make it to the finish line.

Pretty much the only time I say no to sex is when I'm ill, and even then, the line is firmly drawn at stomach issues. If it's just a headache and a mild fever, you might still get lucky (after all, endorphins are the body's natural painkillers), but if there's nausea involved, the jury's out. That's where I say no, and because it happens so infrequently, my husband deems it totally reasonable.

I'm less than two months into this pregnancy, but because I'm spending so much time lying down doing very little, I've had a lot of time to think about all the things I want when it's over and how glorious it will feel to just be tired from regular old sleep deprivation. I know that sounds weird, but I used to have insomnia and average only 4-5 hours sleep a night. It's not great, but at least it's territory I'm familiar with. But I might get lucky. My husband needs less sleep than me, so I might be one of those lucky women that gets to sleep in while their husband deals with the baby at six am. Here's hoping.

Chapter 10- Sick or Pregnant?

Yup, that's the game I've been playing for the last week. I woke up a week ago and felt awful. I mean horrendously awful. Worse than I have for, like, forever! I was feverish, had a splitting headache, and felt seriously queasy, and that lasted for five days. I tried to avoid painkillers for a few days, but after my husband went all science nerd with the scientific journals, I accepted some Tylenol. It helped, but only a bit (and of course, because I'm pregnant I can't take any other medication.)

It began to dawn on me that maybe I wasn't sick. Maybe this was morning sickness. And then I cried, multiple times. Everyone kept reminding me that it would go away after the first twelve weeks but I just wanted to scream, "That's still five weeks away! Make it stop. NOW!" There was no way I was going to be able to survive in that condition for five weeks. It was as if all my worst fears about pregnancy were coming true. I even sobbed to my husband, "Do I really have to do this more than once?" (He'd like more than one kid.)

I tried everything I could to make it better. I had so much ginger that I thought I would turn into a Thai stir fry. I ate protein. I took my vitamins. I smelled peppermint oil. I brushed my teeth when I felt I was going to hurl. I spent more than half of my time in bed. I wore the acupressure bands on my wrists for so long it looked like I'd had them tattooed into my skin when I took them off. I took painkillers. I went for walks. I ate bland foods. Nothing helped.

It's been a week now and I am slightly better, but not completely. Which leads me to believe I was sick but that I probably also now have morning sickness. It just pisses me off. I am always that one in however many people that gets something. ALWAYS. If there's a statistic saying, "One in ten thousand people will find this pill makes them burp pink bubbles," that's me, without fail. But the odds were even less in my favor for this. Apparently 8 out of 10 women get morning sickness.

Why have we, as a species, not evolved to have children in a more pleasant manner? I am seriously annoyed with my baby, which is apparently unusual because most women seem to blame their husbands for making them feel shit, not their baby. It's like my body has been hijacked by someone with no consideration WHATSOEVER for my well-being.

Me: "Uh, baby? Think you could tone it down a bit? Not only do I feel like death, I feel so bad I wish I COULD die."

Baby: "No can do. I'm all happy here. Not gonna change anything."

Me: "Seriously? You are one f***ed up little piece of ****! Just you wait until we reach 9 months! I am going to evict you WITH FORCE and then you'll be sorry! No more cushy living with your fingers on my body controls for you!"

Eventually, after an entire week of total misery, I hauled my sorry ass down to the pharmacy and got some motion sickness pills (check with your doc first if you plan to try this). I took two, immediately, and then walked super slowly home. After half an hour I suddenly felt practically normal. I almost cried. Right there on the street. I was so grateful to not feel as though I was about to lose my guts through my nose at any moment. I can handle fatigue. I cannot handle morning sickness (which, by the way, lasts all day and night, not just in the morning).

I felt so wonderful that I managed to continue on to the store and actually buy something to eat. For the first time in a week, I managed to eat and feel okay. HALELUJA! Forget the ginger and the peppermint. I was cured, with actual drugs. Thank you, medicine. Of course, when I told my best friend I was better because of the pills she asked me, "Are they natural?" I wanted to say that at this point I really don't give a shit if they're natural or not. Besides, as my husband rightly pointed out, "natural" doesn't mean anything. Arsenic is natural, and so is cyanide.

I honestly don't know how women do this more than once. And I honestly don't know how the myth of a "glowing pregnancy" has pervaded when there is SO much evidence to the contrary. Not once have I felt that smug pregnancy satisfaction. All I have felt since I became pregnant was worse than before I was pregnant. It's not exactly endearing me to do this again, so much for survival of the species.

I know everyone tells me it'll be worth it when the baby arrives but... ahem... as I've mentioned before, I don't really like babies. In fact, I even had a conversation with my husband where I told him once the baby is born he's to instruct the doctors/nurses not to plonk it on my chest until it's been cleaned. I know it's supposed to be a bonding moment, but bonding can wait a few minutes. I don't want to be covered in goo thank you very much. Clean it off first.

I have also told my husband that under no circumstances is he allowed below my waist during the birth (assuming it's a natural one). Frankly, I don't think he'll be able to look at my bits the same way again if he sees that. I know it'd freak me out pretty badly to see him push a baby out of his nether regions. I'd certainly get nightmarish flashbacks every time I went down afterwards.

I almost wish births were still like they were when I was born. At my birth, my mum disappeared for a C section and my dad waited in the waiting room. Later, they came out and handed him two clean, wrapped and clothed bundles (me and my twin sister). That's what I'd like. I still want a sex life after this is over so I'd rather not gross out my husband more than is totally necessary. Just drug me up, take the baby out, give it to my husband, and I'll deal with it later when I come back from La La Land.

One thing that struck me about my recent illness was that I was very surprised that my husband didn't get ill too. You see, I went to boarding school, which means I spent 5 years cooped up in a boarding house with 60 other girls. By the end of the 5 years I'd had almost every illness going and had a pretty hefty immune system (only to be outdone by my ex-boyfriend, who also went to boarding school, who had the immune system of a tank and got ill just once in the five years we dated). Normally, if I get ill, my husband gets it too, and when he's ill, he's dying.

So, understandably, I was reasonably suspicious about this illness anomaly, and so off to Google I went. A quick search informed me that I'm far more likely to get ill now that I'm pregnant because my immune system is practically SYSTEM DOWN. Much like with organ transplant medication, in order for my body to not reject the blob growing inside me, my immune system has been slackened so I don't attack the foreign cells inside me.

Great! It's now winter and my immune system is AWOL. Thanks again, baby. Is there anything else I can do for you? Perhaps you'd like my sanity served on a silver platter along with my patience? Now, I've begun to view going out like some sort of bizarre obstacle course. How many door handles and buttons can I avoid touching with my hands? If I'm not careful, I'll turn into my mother, and start wet-wiping everything in sight and running like hell from anyone who sneezes.

One of the most frustrating things now I'm pregnant is that I have to check practically everything I take with a doctor first; vitamins, painkillers, motion sickness pills, supplements… you name it and on the back it either says, "Nope, not for you." Or, "Check with the doctor first." I don't know about you, but I don't have my doctor on speed dial. Can't they just ask a panel of doctors first, and if it isn't safe just say so? Even the most innocuous things I can't take. Like melatonin, to help me sleep. Melatonin is a hormone my own body produces! But I'm not allowed to mess with my own hormone levels. Only the baby is.

It may sound strange, but in a way, I feel a bit violated. Someone has come in, taken over my body, and is now dictating what I'm allowed to do with it. They're making me feel awful, and there's precious little I can do to stop it. Sounds a bit like what would happen if I were being held hostage and interrogated on suspicion of being a spy doesn't it? Despite all the campaigns that a woman's body is her own, I don't feel mine is my own anymore. It's been forcibly taken over with someone else's interests in mind over mine.

My Mother keeps referring to me as "the two of us" but I just don't feel like there's another person inside me yet. It just feels like an inconvenience, not a person. I'd probably find this all a lot easier to cope with if I were attached to "the baby" as if it were a real person, but I'm afraid I just struggle to bond with something that, at this point, looks a lot like a deep-sea fish (i.e. incredibly weird and ugly).

I'm sure my Mother would be horrified to hear me talk like this about my future child (sorry, Mum), but I can't lie. I mostly think this is all weird and annoying. My friends have also reacted in different ways to my current circumstances. One of them is desperate to hear about everything I'm going through in all its gory details, and others I don't talk about it all with, which I'm okay with because I get to pretend nothing's changed. But things have changed, and are about to change very seriously.

Recently I've begun to notice how different my life is now from my friends' on Facebook. I see pictures of them with cocktails, on holidays skiing, or at the beach, I see status updates about their work and dating lives, and I don't do any of those things anymore (to be fair, we live in California so we don't have to go on holiday- we just have to drive to the beach). I'm not really sure who's going to be envious of whom when I have a baby. Will I be envious of their glamorous lives, or will they be envious of my having a settled family? I guess only time will tell.

Chapter 11- Banana Obsessions, Trippy Dreams, Pregnancy Brain, and Olfactory Superpowers

Yup, this week a whole host of pregnancy side effects have come about. After recovering from my illness and apparently curing myself of the most crippling part of my morning sickness, I've begun eating again. However, whereas before I was a complete carnivore, so much so that I'd actually laugh if anyone asked me if I was a vegetarian, I now struggle to eat meat before dinner time.

Vegetables have also become a bit of a problem for me. My husband put some greens before me the other day (normally, I love them) and I suddenly felt exactly like a five-year-old. I was completely turned off by them, and didn't want to touch them. I just scowled at them on my plate and hoped they would magically disappear under my intensely disapproving gaze.

Before all this morning sickness business happened, I could happily eat a pound of meat and ten servings of vegetables in a day. Now I'm lucky if I get one or two servings of greens, and meat isn't happening unless it's almost dinner time. At the moment, all I seem to tolerate well is bananas. Yup, that's it, just bananas. It's like I've become a minion (BANANA!).

I have tried to trick my body by having some vegetables in juice or smoothie form, which has worked, but mostly I seem to be confined to a very narrow range of foods. It's so weird. I dislike things even more than I did as a child. When I was a child there were very few things I didn't like. I didn't like seafood (fish smelled gross), celery (it was all strings so what was the point of it?), mushrooms (yucky texture), and apparently, I didn't like parsnips. But of course, I grew out of those. But now, I've reverted to food preferences that are even more extreme than my own preferences as a kid (except perhaps my strange desire to not have sauces or spreads on anything).

I got an email from my mum the other day reminding me how important it was to eat well and I just wanted to reply that if the baby wanted me to eat well it should stop messing everything up and making that impossible, but I didn't. I just said, "Yes, Mum."

While I'm on the subject of food going in, let's talk about food going out, or not as the case may be. Yes, you guessed it. Another pregnancy side effect is: CONSTIPATION. Oh what joy! As if my innards weren't suffering enough, they've now had a cork stuffed in them, making me look a lot fatter and more pregnant than I am due to the backlog. Something I am less than happy about. Apparently, because my digestive system has "relaxed" due to some hormone the baby is pumping me full of things have gotten a little sluggish.

Oh, and wait… yes. BINGO. You're right again. I'm not allowed to take any laxatives. Of course, I'm not going be bullied by something the size of a raspberry, so, PRUNES to the rescue! I'm not going to sit straining on the toilet until I give myself a hernia. I'm not putting up with that shit (literally). It's coming out one way or another. Take note baby. Two can play at this game.

But on top of all my food preference changes, I've also suddenly developed smelling superpowers. I've always had a fairly good sense of smell, but now it's on a whole different level. It's like I've turned into a dog. I can smell everything, from miles away. This is both good and bad. I can smell my husband's cologne from further away (good) but I can also smell cigarette smoke, sweaty men, and dog poo from miles away (bad).

Just the other day I was walking down the street with my husband when we stopped outside Sephora. He wanted to check if they had my perfume on offer because I'd run out. I took two steps towards the door and froze.

"What's wrong?" my husband asked.

"I can't go in there," I replied. "It's a scent overload! I'll feel sick in about two minutes flat if I go in."

So he went in, and I just stood there on the street slurping my stealthy vegetable smoothie.

I always used to find some stores off limits to me, like Lush and Abercrombie & Fitch, because they pumped out enough perfume to knock out a small rhinoceros. But now, even more places seem to be off limits. I'm also finding I'm sneezing a lot more because scents are getting to me more these days. I pretty much cross the street to avoid smokers now, and I can't talk to someone if they've been eating something that makes me feel queasy if I can smell it on their breath (which makes for some rather abrupt conversations).

The next thing I noticed was that I'm suddenly terribly thirsty like, ALL THE TIME! I can drink ten big glasses of water during the day, be so hydrated that my pee is the same color as the toilet water, and I still wake up in the middle of the night parched, with lips so cracked you'd think I'd just crawled out of the desert. Other than taking up residence in an aquarium, there's no way I could consume more water, but no matter how much I drink, it just never seems to be enough.

Of, course, off to Dr. Google I went, who informed me that I wasn't turning into a fish, but my blood volume was increasing and in order to accommodate that, my blood vessels were dilating, meaning I was letting off more heat than I ordinarily would have. This had the side effect of meaning I was hot stuff (literally- I'm too hot for my husband to hug at night in bed) so I was losing more water sweating in an effort to keep my cool.

However, like I said, I'm not taking this pregnancy thing sitting down (well, I am actually, but you know what I mean in a metaphorical sense). My husband happens to be the creator of a cooling vest. It was originally designed for weight loss (it chills you and forces you to burn calories as heat) but seeing as I'm already about as hot as the surface of the sun, all it does is keep me cool (very effectively I might add- coldsh.com for anyone who cares to check it out).

And now let's get to the last, most wacko pregnancy side effect this week: MENTAL DREAMS. I mean crazy vivid dreams that have no foundation in logic at all. Every time I wake up in the night I wake up from an extremely clear, weird dream. The only good thing about this is that my husband finds it terribly funny to hear about them in the morning. I'll give you a few examples, just for your own amusement.

I was working in a fancy restaurant as the hostess and it was a big night, opening night or something. Halfway through the dinner service an important chef from another restaurant came in. He sat at the bar and looked at the menu. When the waiter came to take his order, he got very cross that there were no "rapid" dishes he could order (dishes that would come out super-fast). The waiter apologized and suggested he have the oysters as they were quick to prepare. The chef agreed and asked if they had any chili for them. The waiter said no, but they had tomato. The chef then went totally mental saying you never put tomato with oysters. I remember thinking, "I must tell the owner we shouldn't put tomato with the oysters."

This dream was nuts because not only have I never worked in a restaurant, I know jack shit about oysters. I have no idea why you would or wouldn't put tomato with them and I know for a fact I wouldn't want to work as a hostess because I like to work during the day and then go to bed at night. But

49

compared to some of my other dreams, this was on the tame side.

In a dream I had last night, I was with a group and we were running away from some people. We ran to a safe house that was situated on a cliff by the coast. We hid inside and I looked out the window. I could see the sea and the small beach cove below. However, after a moment I noticed there were some people swimming towards us. One of them was Draco Malfoy from *Harry Potter*, one was Jamie Laing from *Made in Chelsea*, and the other I couldn't see. I ran to the front door to lock us in but they were already there. Then I realized the third person was my ex-boyfriend's younger brother, (who is totally non-violent in real life). He proceeded to try and kick the door in and I managed to lock it just in time. Then I woke up.

And in one of my more zany dreams I was sneaking around involved in some sort of covert ops, avoiding puffs of purple smoke. However, that theme didn't last very long. Before I knew it, I was in a room with another girl and we were being interrogated by Matthew McConaughey for a beauty contest. He noted that we were the only two girls he'd seen so far who hadn't smoked. I asked how he knew and he said he'd seen the other girls smoking near the emergency room of a hospital I used to live near in London. I figured he'd only know where that was if he lived there too. So I asked him. He coyly didn't answer but admitted he'd worked at the Waitrose (an upmarket British supermarket) up the road but had quit because the pay was rubbish. Then I woke up with my husband asking me if I wanted a cup of tea.

I have to say, out of all the pregnancy side effects, the weird dreams are by far the coolest and least intrusive on my body. I really don't care how far my brain goes into LSD dream territory, as long as the rest of me feels normal (which unfortunately, isn't happening). I also feel like I'm getting more forgetful that I was before. Or perhaps careless is the right way to describe it. I'm forgetting to bring things to places, walking out of stores without a key ingredient for a recipe, and putting things down where I shouldn't.

Just the other day I was eating in the kitchen (woo hoo- I managed to eat!) when I heard my husband swear violently next door. I rushed through to see if he was okay. He was, but when I went back in the kitchen I found my fork, piece of steak attached, on the countertop just a few inches away from my plate. I know it may sound like a minor thing, but I've never done something like that before. I would never put my steak on the countertop. NEVER. But here I am, carelessly throwing things down anywhere.

I googled "pregnancy brain" and it appears to be a real thing. Women get stupider when pregnant. I suppose it's because our body is busy with more important things than thinking (doesn't that sound like something a 1950's man would say?) And while I was at it, I also consulted Google on what pregnancy was like for the significant other in the relationship. I honestly don't know why I did, but I typed in "Why is my pregnant wife so..." Want to know what Google suggested for the next words? The top two hits were: mean and moody.

Now, I suppose I could be biased here, but I don't feel I've gotten very moody since becoming pregnant. In fact, I asked my husband if I have (yes, that's dangerous territory for him but he's never been shy of giving his real opinion, sometimes to his detriment). He said I wasn't moody but there'd been more tears than usual because I cry when I feel really unwell. I just feel sorry for myself. I loathe feeling nauseous.

So, seeing as I usually get every side effect under the sun but hadn't gotten this one I was understandably curious as to why so many women were apparently turning into psychopaths but I wasn't. I read a few of the blogs and the comments from men underneath and was genuinely sad about what they had to say. Some of them said their wives would scream at them, say nasty things, and even be physically violent towards them. And, of course, all the women were blaming it on "hormones."

Now, I'm aware that there are some hormonal conditions (such as a really bad form of PMS) that are medically recognized as turning you into a murderous psychopath, and for those women I really do sympathize because their behavior is basically out of their control. However, I have a sneaking suspicion that many women could be unconsciously making their mood swings worse and simply blaming it all on hormones.

Let's re-visit my previous rant about how I feel pregnant women often just use being pregnant as an excuse to eat whatever they want. What are the things that women often want to eat but would never normally allow in huge quantities? Chocolate, chips, cookies, crackers, bread, pizza, ice cream, biscuits... basically any refined form of sugar. Why do I feel women are unconsciously making their moods worse with this? Regardless of pregnancy, there is a well-established link between sugar and mood swings.

Everyone knows the phrases "sugar high" and "sugar crash." We all feel giddy with sugar where everything is great and then we crash, and are depressed, irritable, and often mean. Now... imagine adding that on top of your already fluctuating hormone levels. What do you think might happen? KABOOM! We have a TNT on PMS hormonal situation.

I'm well aware that there are some women out there screaming, "But I'm so sick that's all I can eat! How dare you judge me! You don't know what it's like!" Actually, I do. I've felt very sick for a while now too. In fact, I spent an entire week basically only being able to eat ripe bananas (they had to be ripe!). I could have gone back on the refined carbs, but I didn't want to because they wouldn't have been good for my body. So I found something else that I could tolerate. Something that would give my blood sugar a boost, but something that also had fiber and would help stabilize my blood sugar levels to avoid that sugar crash.

I don't pretend to be a dietary expert, but I am prepared to say that if your partner feels you've turned into a homicidal maniac, you may want to consider ditching the fast sugar in a bid to save your relationship from serious damage. From the posts I read, the men were either terrified or seriously considering leaving. Yes, we're the ones going through all the pain, but your partner isn't superman. You can't go all psycho on them and expect them to cope perfectly. They're only human (and even superman has a chink in his armor: kryptonite).

And for the record, how we pregnant women feel is NOT your partner's fault. It's the baby's fault. Let's not confuse where the blame lies here. We are 50:50 responsible with our partners for the baby being there (it takes two to tango) but it's the baby's fault you feel like crap. They are the one doing a hostile takeover of your body. Don't take it out on your scared partner. Bar the odd exception, all your partner wants is to help you and for you to feel better. Don't bite their head off.

Chapter 12– Flying High in the First Trimester

Nope, I'm not talking about feeling high. I'm talking about being literally high, in a plane. Yes, I am just getting over having flown across the Atlantic to see my parents. I'm not the best of travelers, but normally I travel okay. I may feel ill but I'm never actually sick. I'm also a notoriously bad sleeper on planes, trains, or anything that requires me to remain upright. The general rule is: if I can't lie down, sleep won't happen.

Flying in the first trimester isn't really risky from a health standpoint. It's far more risky to fly in your last trimester. So much so that some airlines won't take you as a passenger because of the risk you might go into labor and they'll have to make an emergency stop which would mess up their flight schedule and inconvenience an entire plane-load of passengers who don't give a shit about your newly acquired bundle of joy. They care about getting to their destination on time.

This time, I didn't leave anything to chance on my flight. I took motion sickness pills beforehand (which I haven't needed when travelling since I was very little). I brought a bag of crystallized ginger. I worse my sea bands, and I chose a seat at the very back of the plane. I did that for two reasons. On Virgin planes, if you sit at the back you can recline your seat as far as you want without pissing anyone off (not all airlines let back row seats recline- check individual airlines). Plus, sitting at the very back greatly increased my chances of getting a second seat to myself, and I did.

Smugly happy with my preparations and two seats, I thought things were going my way. What a laughable notion. The plane was 40 minutes late leaving and we had one of the worst take offs and initial flights I've ever had. The turbulence was horrendous. I ended up pressing on my acupressure bands so hard I thought my hands might fall off. I've rarely felt worse. Given that I was already rather prone to feeling queasy under the best of conditions, it was frankly a miracle that my dinner didn't make a second appearance.

I then spent the next six or so hours doing what looked like a mixture of yoga and origami in an effort to find at least a semi-comfortable position to sleep in. I managed to curl up flat on my two seats, but it was hardly comfortable. So, I only got about four hours of sleep tops (which is actually better than normal for me on a plane). Luckily, there were some good films to watch and bizarrely I felt pretty good for the rest of the day once I landed. Then I woke up the next morning.

I can't really think of any other way to describe it except that jet lag and morning sickness go together like death metal and Barbie. Not only is your body rather confused about when it should feel sick (mine seemed to just decide to cover all bases and feel crap 24/7) but the exhaustion and general "icky" feeling you get from regular jet lag seems to exacerbate all symptoms of morning sickness.

I spent almost a week practically skipping every morning. Staying in bed until at least 10:30 and then having to wear my sea bands round the clock and take motion sickness pills even though I wasn't moving anymore while I attempted to eat something and not just collapse into a pathetic puddle on the floor. It built up in severity until yesterday. I lost the battle. I was sick, for real. Luckily, the house was empty and I had no witnesses to the sorry affair.

One of the things I hate the most about being sick is that everything runs. Not only is my food coming back for an encore, my nose starts to run, and tears stream down my face. The only good thing about it was that I felt a lot better afterwards. Today I have managed to avoid a repeat episode, which I am very thankful for because I can't afford to lose any more food options right now.

Usually, if I've been ill after eating something in particular, I can't touch that food again for at least a significant while, if ever. I can't eat coronation chicken, Nutella, or porridge for that reason. And right now, my food options are so limited that I'd be eating air if I lost any. However, I am hoping that soon this trauma will end. By the end of this week I'll be 10 weeks pregnant and I'm praying my stomach will settle at 12, for good.

One of the other side effects I seem to have randomly developed since arriving on this side of the pond is night sweats. Without fail, I wake up at around 5am drenched in sweat. I'm wet, the sheets are wet, and everything is sticky. I know I don't have too many covers on because for the rest of the night I'm only just warm enough. I don't know why my body has chosen to treat my bed like a sauna at 5am, but it has. All I can manage is to lift up the covers until I dry off. I certainly can't be bothered to get up and shower at that ungodly hour.

In some ways, it has been nice to be back with my parents. I have been able to ask my Mother a bit about her pregnancies, and my parents have been pretty understanding of my uselessness. My Mother is funny though. No sooner had I plonked my bag down in my room than I noticed there were pregnancy books and leaflets everywhere. I don't remember us having owned them before, so she must have picked them up before I came. To be honest, I haven't really read them yet. I still find the pictures a bit off putting. Anything that has a 1:1 ratio of head to body is a weird thing in my mind.

I met up with my best friend the other day and she asked me whether I felt I'd bonded with the baby. I immediately answered with a flat out "no." I don't feel attached to it at all. In fact, I don't really feel like there's a person growing in me. I just feel sick, like I have some terrible cold or something. Not once have I patted my stomach or talked to it (other than right after I was sick when I begged it to knock it off!)

My best friend, like most people, is far more excited about me being pregnant than I am. We passed a store with a child's mannequin in the window and she squealed, "If you have a girl you can dress her like that!" At this point, all my energy is focused on just getting to a point where I feel better. I'm not thinking any further ahead than waking up and being able to get up and have breakfast, and it tasting great.

On the subject of my best friend, one of the reasons we're over in the UK this Christmas is to have a UK wedding blessing for my UK side of the family (we got married in the U.S. earlier this year). Of course, my best friend wouldn't accept my excuse for not having a hen do (I'm already married) and forced one on me last weekend. To be fair to her, for the most part it was great. We had afternoon tea and dinner out in London, which were fine, but she also forced a burlesque class on me. She loved it, and it was kind of fun, but it's almost impossible to feel sexy in the early stages of pregnancy. There I was, peeling my stockings off, wishing I could lie down in the pile of feather boas for a nap.

In a way, seeing my friends really did hammer home how different we are now. They're becoming lawyers, starting their own companies, training to be professors, and here I am: married and pregnant. I am working on my dream of becoming a writer, but as far as my friends can see, I'm a pregnant housewife. But there's something dirty about the word "housewife" these days. It somehow implies you have no ambition and you're merely taking it easy while your partner brings home the bacon.

I spoke to my dad after my hen do because my best friend and I seriously disagreed over a topic at dinner. I simply do not believe you can have it all. In my opinion, it's impossible to have a high-flying career, be at home with your kids, and have a great relationship with your partner. She thought you could have it all, and told me she knows two executives that work part time and do have it all (somehow, I think behind the scenes they don't).

My dad said something very interesting. He said men can't have it all either. He said men sacrifice seeing much of their children's lives to be at work and earn money, but by the woman taking on a stay-at-home role, they are able to focus on work, and do well at it, therefore bringing home a good salary. He said when women and men try to share the work and parenting duties, it all tends to go to pot. It's a nice idea, but not one that realistically plays out that well.

I suppose some people might say his view is old fashioned, but I'm inclined to agree with him. I really don't believe women can have it all if by "having it all" we mean a high-powered job, a great relationship, and the ability to raise children in a yummy mummy fashion. If you have a high-powered job, you'll have a nanny or day care. If you raise your children yourself and have a great relationship, you won't have time for a high-powered job. If you have a high-powered job and try to be a yummy mummy, you won't have time left over for your partner. The way I see it, you get two out of the three.

The workplace is not friendly to mums. You can disagree with me all you like, but I've seen the dread and eye rolls male managers give when their female staff get pregnant. Women going on maternity leave are highly disruptive to most workplaces. Saying it's not an issue is like saying sexism in banking isn't an issue. Realistically, having kids does affect your career.

Now, I'm not saying women can't work at all. They can. But having a 9-5 (or 9-6 as is often the case) job is, in my opinion, out of the question if you actually want to raise your own children. A job with flexible hours or freelance work is much more realistic. Besides, who wouldn't rather work from home? Screw the commute! You can work in your pajamas from home.

Chapter 13- Tears and Tantrums

Yes, that's right. I've finally lost my cool and perhaps this time I actually get to blame it on pregnancy hormones. In my defense, it took two and a half weeks of my Mother's fussing before I cracked. So what was the catalyst? Perhaps, unsurprisingly, my Mother was the catalyst. I know she only meant well, but it was beyond what I could handle at the time. What did my Mother do that was so bad? She went through my room at my parent's house, tidying it up, found the replacement motion sickness pills I'd bought in the UK to replace the American ones I'd been taking, called the pharmacist behind my back and told me I wasn't allowed to take the UK ones anymore because they weren't safe.

Let's first address the issue of whether the pills I was taking were safe. As far as I and my scientist husband were concerned, they were safe. They were a slightly newer version of motion sickness pills than what was available in the U.S. Therefore, extensive testing had not been done on them. However, there was nothing to say they WEREN'T safe. But just to be sure, lawyers insist on plonking the label "not to be taken by pregnant women unless advised by a doctor" on everything not extensively tested. It's a legal cover-your-ass type thing. However, this was not a good enough argument for my Mother and she insisted I shouldn't take them. So, I burst into violent tears.

Why did I get so upset? Part of it was probably hormones, but I actually have a tendency to cry when I feel unwell, pregnant or not. And I got THAT upset because she was telling me not to take the ONLY thing that was making my life bearable. I wept and spluttered that in reality, I wasn't doing fine (we Brits like to pretend all is fine even when it's not – stiff upper lip and all that). I sobbed that I felt awful ALL THE TIME. I even uttered the words, "No one cares about me. All anyone cares about is how the baby is doing. What about me?! Why should I have to suffer this much? According to a pharmacist I'm not even allowed to take a bloody laxative! I'm just supposed to stay bunged up until I explode! If I had known it would be this bad I would never have gotten pregnant in the first place and I'd rather have an abortion than go through this again!"

<Sharp intake of breath> Yes, I really said that. And no, it wasn't just the hormones talking. I really felt that bad that I really meant (at that moment) what I said about the abortion. My Mother was slightly taken aback by my seemingly out of the blue outburst. She said she'd felt ill too when pregnant but clearly not as bad as I did (I certainly don't remember her being bedbound or sick when she was pregnant with my brother). She hugged me and assured me we'd go to the doctor and sort it out. Apparently, the only person she would listen to about the pills was a doctor. So, I agreed to go and limped up to my room to my very surprised husband.

"What's wrong?" he asked.

Between sobs I managed to splutter out an explanation and he burst out laughing. Clearly, he wasn't particularly concerned about the matter, but he researched the UK pills and did his best to explain to my Mother that he was happy with me taking them and he felt they didn't pose a risk to me. Did my Mother listen to my husband, the pedantic scientist? No, of course not!

The next morning I came down to breakfast, or rather, to a glass of full sugar coke to squash my nausea, to be informed that we were going to a private doctor nearby because the NHS doctors couldn't see me that day. I had to say, it did rather put a spanner in my plans for the day because I was supposed to be making my wedding cake for the wedding blessing at the weekend, for which we were leaving the next day. But I learned a long time ago that there was no point trying to reason my side with my Mother. It was easier to just agree. She wasn't going to listen to anyone but a doctor (okay, a medical doctor – apparently my husband's PhD didn't count). So, despite the cake duties backlogging, I acquiesced, and off we went.

The doctor was a nice man and because it was a private doctor, I got a 30-minute appointment with him. However, most of the appointment was filled with my Mother's questions:

Mum: "I'm worried she's still anemic."
Doctor: "Her blood pressure is fine, her pulse is fine, and there's no sign of anemia from her eyes."
Mum: "But she should still have a blood test to check?"
Doctor: "To be safe, yes. But there are no obvious signs."
Mum: "And these pills, are they safe?"
Doctor: <Online research and book flipping> "There's nothing to say they're not

safe but I'll prescribe something else for you that's cheaper."

Mum: "So you'll give her something else?"

Doctor: "Yes. She can take these if she wants but it's better value for money to get a prescription for a greater quantity of something."

Mum: "And what about her diet? She doesn't eat lots of foods. Is she deficient?"

Me: "I believe I have Celiac Disease and I don't eat any grains because it's like a grenade goes off in my stomach when I do. I also don't eat any nightshades or dairy because they don't agree with me."

Mum: "But should she be eating these? Could she be giving the baby sensitivities by avoiding these foods?"

Me: <Outraged look>

Doctor: "The baby is quite protected in the womb, so if these foods cause negative reactions, she probably shouldn't have them."

And on it went. We left, prescription in hand, with my Mother feeling greatly reassured. We had essentially paid to have her worries calmed by a doctor. We got the prescription for a type of anti-histamine and went home.

The first chance I had to try the new medication was on the morning of the wedding blessing, because I couldn't find my other ones. Without going into gory detail, it's sufficient to say they didn't work. I spent half an hour on the floor trying not to move lest I hurl before texting my sister begging someone to bring me a coke (yes, sugary coke really does kill nausea for a while). She called room service and the woman who brought it told me it was probably nerves (I was in the bridal suite). I agreed because I didn't want to spend time explaining my situation. I wanted the coke.

Eventually, I mustered the courage to get off the floor and get dressed. I also found my real medication and took that as soon as I could. It was going to be a busy day and I didn't have time to spare with my head hanging over the toilet bowl. I had a wedding dress and an act to put on. After all, most of the guests didn't know I was pregnant, so I had no real excuse to be poorly. The dress went on, the make-up went on, and the smile went on.

The wedding day turned out fine, and when we got back my husband's emergency Amazon order of more American motion sickness pills had arrived. So, I went back to those, for my Mother's sanity, and I suppose, in turn, for mine too because she apparently hadn't been listening when the doctor said the UK pills I'd been taking were fine, because she couldn't recall him saying that at all. All she'd heard was, "I'll prescribe something else." <Sigh>

Chapter 14– Bye Bye Morning Sickness, Hello Ravenous Appetite

Houston, we have reached 12 weeks. I AM CURED! THE MORNING SICKNESS IS GONE! I have rarely been so grateful for anything in my life. I'm serious. I'm even more grateful than when my university exams were over. I'm just so elated to feel normal, for my stomach to feel settled. It's utter bliss and it couldn't have been more timely because we're flying back to California in a few days and I don't think I can endure another rough flight. My last flight was complete hell what with the morning sickness and turbulence.

I just got so fed up of everything morning sickness related. I swear there are still indents in my arms from the sea bands and I honestly don't think I'll ever be able to eat ginger again. I've been pavlovian trained to associate it with prayers for someone to end my queasy misery. Ginger ale? No thank you!

What's more, the morning sickness isn't the only thing that seems to have gotten better at the 12-week mark. Suddenly my ultra-sensitive boobs feel almost normal again. I mean, they're still huge, watermelon sized (but I've gotten used to that), but they no longer hurt so much anymore. My husband can actually hug me properly again and I can lie on my stomach to sleep without wincing.

Speaking of sleep, I'm also now able to sleep for more than two hours without having to get up to use the bathroom too. Previously, it was like clockwork, every two hours. Now I can go three or four hours between bathroom trips. Woo hoo! Small victories count to the sleep deprived. Google informs me that this is because my uterus has moved forward, relieving the pressure on my bladder (yeah, I'll enjoy that while it lasts).

However, these improvements haven't been without new symptoms to replace them. Say goodbye to nausea, food aversions, and constant bathroom trips, and hello to headaches, dizziness, and eyeing up anything left on anyone's plate. I'm not joking about the last one either. I am a lot hungrier than I was before. I don't know whether it's my body trying to catch up after the morning sickness, or whether my appetite has just seriously kicked up a gear, but I am a lot hungrier.

However, what with my previous rants about pregnant women over-eating, I have been trying to watch what I eat. Now before you get outraged, let me make this clear. I am not on a diet. I don't count calories (too much math), but I have been trying to keep my somewhat increased food intake to healthy foods (not hard when there's a lot of leftover turkey from Christmas in the house- lean meat).

I have loved being back in the UK from a food point of view. There is all this food that I can eat that I couldn't buy in the U.S. because they put stuff in it I couldn't eat. Here, I've been able to eat salami that didn't contain wheat or dairy. One pound fifty would buy me a packet of salami with no crap in it. And I certainly took advantage of that. And just being able to walk into a supermarket and pick up a packet of lunch meat that didn't have an ingredient list as long as my arm has been wonderful. It makes eating on the go so much easier.

In fact, my husband sent me an email with a link saying we're only going to eat organic in the U.S. from now on because he was worried about the fertilizers they use and their effects on developing children. It is a sad fact that the food standards (both in taste, quality, and safety) are a lot higher in Europe. So, I guess we'll be frequenting the farmer's markets more.

I am really enjoying being able to eat more normally. All my food aversions are gone and even my cravings seem to have disappeared. Whilst at my parents' house I developed a sudden obsession with mushrooms. I wanted them in everything. There were no pickles and ice cream cravings for me. I just wanted mushrooms, and lots of them. The only explanation I could think of was that I was low on vitamin D, what with England being such a grey place and all.

Now my diet has practically returned to what it was pre-pregnancy, lots of vegetables, meat, fish, and some fruit. That may sound boring to some, and my Mother certainly questioned it, but my husband was happy to point out that in fact, he thinks I eat healthier than almost everyone. Mind you, around Christmas when everyone was stuffing themselves with chocolate and gingerbread, it wasn't a hard accolade to achieve. So, I'm not too smug about it.

I may feel more normal now but the only person in my family who isn't treating me any different now that I'm pregnant is my sixteen-year-old brother.

Perhaps it's just because he's young, but nothing seems to have changed at all as far as he's concerned. When he asks me about me, he really means me. He's not asked a single question about my pregnancy, and I'm glad.

I've always felt that women seem to disappear when they become Mothers, and I'd always assumed it was their own fault, but all of a sudden I've begun to feel as though I'm disappearing, because that's how everyone is treating me. I feel as though people can't see beyond my growing stomach, and everything is related to the baby.

For example, the other night I was in the kitchen with my brother and we were comparing boy's names for a character in a story I was writing. We had written a few down and were trying to narrow it down. EVERYONE who came into the kitchen immediately assumed I was trying to pick baby names.

Okay, firstly, I'm not going to bother picking baby names until I know the sex of the baby. Why would you make your life harder by choosing names for both genders when you don't have to? Secondly, I would have thought it was obvious from the types of names on our list that they were not something I would choose for my baby. I'm not likely to name a child Milo or Tobias when they're likely going to grow up in California. Milo works in Chelsea, not Laguna Beach.

It's just getting annoying, I've finally started to feel normal and people are treating me as though I've been replaced by a baby making machine with no goals of its own. I just feel like saying, "Hello! I'm still here!" Other than the trauma I'm going through, I actually have no interest in my pregnancy. As long as everything is developing as it's supposed to, I'm not interested in reading up on what's going on inside me. The books can keep their creepy pictures because I'm just not interested.

Chapter 15- Jet Lag's a Bitch

Okay, so I'm back in the U.S. and the trip was only marginally easier than the last one. In fact, I'd go so far as to say I felt significantly worse when I landed (but at least there wasn't any turbulence). We flew back Norwegian Air which was a perfectly good airline. In fact, they'd made several modifications to their planes help with jet lag. The plane was pressurized to a lower altitude and there was more oxygen in the air. They also had some funky LED lighting so you weren't blinded by the sun out of the window.

However, none of this really mattered because a few rows behind me was a baby, a screaming baby. Now, that was totally fine for say, the first seven hours, but after that I desperately needed some sleep and I COULD NOT GET IT! The baby did not stop. Even with earplugs I could hear it yelling and the only way to drown it out was with music or a film, but I can't sleep with noise like that on.

I know I shouldn't be criticizing seeing as I'll soon be in that parent's position, but knowing that didn't change my body's perspective on the matter. My exhausted, pregnant body was screaming out for sleep and I simply couldn't get any for the ear shattering noise coming from behind me. It got so bad that I actually started crying I was so tired (did you know you can cry with your eyes closed?). The last time I cried in public due to exhaustion was at Heathrow baggage claim after my flight from Nairobi had been delayed until 2am and then I'd gotten no sleep because a fat woman's thighs had been taking up half my seat.

I tried my best to be understanding, but all I wanted to do was run away from the noise or scream, "Shove a boob in its mouth, damnnit! At least muffle it will ya?" But, being British, I said nothing. I just sat in my seat and silently cried until we landed. I think the man next to me picked up on it because when we were leaving the plane he held up foot traffic to let me out and helped me get my bag down. I knew he just felt sorry for me, but hey, I wasn't going to turn down pity that enabled me to get off the plane faster.

Both my husband and I were shattered. So much so that we didn't even make it home from the airport. We gave up about 20 minutes away and checked into a hotel. In our defense, the new house was totally empty. We would have had to assemble the bed before we could have slept. We fell into bed at 7pm and didn't move until 4am. It was heaven. Good hotels have the best soundproofing and the fluffiest beds. After my squashed, noisy plane trip, I couldn't have been happier.

The next morning, however, we were presented with a slight problem. You see, what with me being pregnant, breakfast is a rather urgent matter. And with jet lag, it's even worse, because the nausea comes back unless I put some food into my system PRONTO! And we scrambled to leave in a hurry before I started to heave. Luckily, with it being an American hotel and all, we found a coke vending machine in the hallway, and crisis temporarily averted, we checked out.

We ended up stopping for breakfast at an IHOP (International House of Pancakes) because it was the only place I could think of that I knew was open 24 hours a day. Why did I know that? It was in some song lyric. "Open all night like an IHOP." I had actually never been to an IHOP before. There are lots of typically American things that I've never done and many that I will never do due to my food issues. I've never had a Krispy Kreme doughnut, I've never been to a Taco Bell, I've never had a Twinkie, and I've never been to a frozen yogurt chain (which seems to be all the rage at the moment).

The IHOP was perfectly nice but seeing as I couldn't eat any of the pancake type things, I just ordered a few sides of fruit and meat to go with my tea and stared out of the dark window at the town that was to be my new home. I'm not quite sure how I feel about living in true suburbia. I mean, it's boring but the beach is ten minutes away. And sometimes boring is good. It allows you to get on with other things you've been neglecting because you were too easily distracted.

We've now been in the new house for a week and we've barely unpacked beyond the essentials. I've spent the vast majority of the last week asleep and my husband has spent most of his time catching up on work stuff. But I am finally over my jet lag (thank God) and am starting to contemplate what to do with the house. But before you get excited, no, I'm not thinking about a nursery.

We're actually going to be renting the other two rooms of our house out for the rest of my pregnancy (why wouldn't you?) and even after that, I don't think we'll bother with a nursery for a while. You see, American houses are HUGE.

There's a walk-through wardrobe thing between our room and the bathroom/rest of the house, so I reckon we'll eventually just plonk the crib in there. After all, why would you want to walk further than you have to in the middle of the night?

I haven't seen anyone we know since we've gotten back. We've been too busy, so I don't think news of my pregnancy has really spread. But sooner or later it will become obvious to people. Speaking of me becoming obvious, I didn't have time to sort out an ultrasound in the UK, so I'm booked in to have my first scan this week. I don't really want to see something growing inside me, to be honest, but I do want to know whether I have one or two clingers on.

My concerns about the possibility of me carrying twins are not unfounded. I have a twin sister and my Mother's brother and sister are twins. And before any of you start, no, non-identical twins do not skip a generation, and to be honest that sounds like an old wives' tale anyway. In a way, I actually want it to be twins, that way I won't have to go through this again. What's more, they'll always have someone to play with.

Booking my scan appointment was a slightly odd experience. Everyone keeps saying, "Congratulations!" as if I've achieved some sort of Nobel Prize. The doctor on the phone said it too but I don't think my rather sarcastically British response of, "Thanks, but I didn't do much," really went down too well. What I really wanted to say was, "Thanks, but I didn't do anything but spread my legs, but I'll pass the compliment on to my ovaries." However, I figured that'd be a step too far for the American sense of humor. So, I kept that remark to myself.

I just have this feeling that the doctors here aren't going to know what to do with me because I'm not the classic excited pregnant woman about to cry at seeing her baby for the first time. I'm more like the, "Great, that's all very nice but please get to the point. Is everything fine or not? I have other things to do today like work out the decor for my bathroom."

I've also decided that I may have to buy a few more maternity clothes because my wardrobe is like a bad mood grenade waiting to go off. Every time I try to wear something I used to like and I see how badly it now fits I get really annoyed. So, to spare everyone a tantrum, I think a little shopping is in order. There's not a huge variety of choice for pregnant women (I mean, there's only so many ways you can dress up a tent), but I'm sure I'll be able to find something I don't hate.

The only problem about searching for anything baby related online is that

Google remembers your searches, so all the adverts that pop up are to do with babies. I've recently gotten really annoyed with YouTube constantly showing me a Clearblue ovulation test advert. It's like, "Fuck off! I don't need that. I'm already pregnant! Stop showing me pictures of cute babies when I know full well they only look cute 20% of the time. The other 80% they're either screaming or unnervingly staring at you."

I'm also trying to get to grips with my increased need for sleep and food. As in, if I don't get food within 15 minutes of me saying I'm hungry, I get pretty cranky, and if I don't get enough sleep, I turn into a zombie. My husband is also trying to adjust to the newfound urgency of these two things. We had a minor tiff in a department store the other day because I had said I was hungry but he disappeared to look for shirts. Needless to say, when I found him we left to get food and the shopping was done afterwards.

I guess that's another reason I want to know if I'm carrying twins or not. It would definitely explain why I'm so hungry at this early stage. I'm only three months pregnant, after all. I shouldn't need to be stuffing my face yet. But at the moment, if I don't eat every 4 hours, it's not good. I've always had the theory that the fashion world is so bitchy because hungry people are angry people, and my current experience is only acting to confirm those suspicions.

I am aware that some weight gain is an inevitable part of pregnancy, and for that very reason I have refused to step on the scales since my positive pregnancy test. My boobs have inflated, my blood volume has increased, and my uterus is growing with increasing fluid. There's no way I WON'T put on weight. But I'm trying not to but on too much fat. A couple pounds is probably okay as I'll be able to lose that again fairly quickly, but I really don't want to put on much more fat than that.

I can't pretend I'm not upset by my changing body. I am upset that my stomach is getting bigger and my boobs still seem to be growing. I'm not even kidding. The bras I bought a month ago are seriously snug now, and in fact, one of the straps on them broke under the sheer weight of my boob. That's right! My boob weight broke the bra strap. Of course, when I told my husband this I didn't get any sympathy. He simply said, "THAT. IS. AWESOME!"

Chapter 16— That Blob is Your Baby

This morning I had my first checkup and ultrasound. It was at the somewhat unspeakable hour of 8am, meaning I had to get up at 6:30 (because I can't skip breakfast these days). Let me first just say, the amount of paperwork you have to do to see a doctor in the U.S. is just ridiculous. I had, like, ten sheets to fill out!

After the mountain of paperwork was done a doctor appeared and said, "We'll do your ultrasound now." I had been told I would have to come back at 11am for the ultrasound after I'd seen the nurse at 8am, but I suppose that's one of the benefits of being the first appointment. They can squeeze you in before anyone else arrives.

We followed the doctor to a room and she asked me to strip from the waist down. Having had several IUD insertions over the years, I wasn't freaked out by this, but she still left to let me change in private (even though she would shortly be getting a good look at my privates). My husband just sat in the chair with a smug look on his face at the unexpected striptease.

After a few minutes the doctor returned and asked me to lie down. I did, and that was when I noticed I had an audience. They'd stuck a picture on the ceiling of four cats staring down curiously, presumably to cheer you up if you were nervous (which I was). It definitely worked. Cats, in my opinion, pretty much always improve any situation. The funniest videos on the internet are always of cats, cats and children, in that order.

The doctor asked me if I had any concerns (I told her it could be twins given my family history), covered my stomach with blue goo, and proceeded to prod around. At first, we couldn't really see anything on the massive TV monitor on the wall (it's America - everything is big) but then something baby shaped came into view.

"It's definitely just one," she said. "Not twins."

I wasn't really sure if I was happy about that news or not. I had been a bit worried about how huge I would have become with twins, but I had also hoped that if it had been twins, I wouldn't ever have to be pregnant again and endure the crippling sickness and fatigue (and massive boobs) that came along with it.

True to family traits, my baby wasn't being very cooperative. It was moving lots, so much so that my husband said, "Can you not feel that? It's bouncing around like it's going to be a figure skater!" but it wasn't in the right position to take certain measurements. So, the doctor prodded and poked with the ultrasound machine, asked me to lie this way and that, tried getting a better view with the vaginal ultrasound (which my husband later referred to as "the dildo ultrasound"), but my baby defiantly stayed upside down.

"We'll have to scan you again after you see the nurse," she said. "You baby's a little troublemaker already."

"Can you tell the gender at this stage?" my husband asked.

"Oh sure," the doctor replied. "Did you want to know?"

We exchanged a brief glance before both saying, "Yes."

"It's a girl."

I have to say, both my husband and I were fairly unemotional about the whole thing. Neither of us was too excited about seeing the baby for the first time and there was no squealing or tears when we heard the heartbeat. However, my husband did have a fairly big grin on his face afterwards. So, I suspect he was a bit excited about it. I, unfortunately, felt a little indifferent.

Much like how I had mixed feelings about it not being twins, I had mixed feelings about it being a girl, only because I know what a pain girls can be, especially as teenagers. Without wanting to stereotype too much, boys tend to be a little more straightforward than girls. They say what they mean and their thought patterns don't tend to be over-complicated.

Apparently, I wasn't a very difficult baby, and as a child, I was a tomboy and did boy things, like play with toy cars, climb trees, and do DIY with my Father. So, my daughter could turn out like that. On the other hand, she could turn out like my sister, who was a much fussier child. I remember clearly passing my sister's room aged 4 or 5 to hear her throwing a tantrum because her favorite underwear wasn't clean and she wouldn't wear anything else but those.

The scope for unreasonable behavior seems to be larger with girls, but I guess I'll just have to wait and see how far on the crazy scale my daughter ranks. And whilst I know I'm not really in control, I would prefer it if my next child was a boy. Two teenage girls in one house isn't something I particularly want to go through (having been one of two teenage girls in a house).

After the first scan was over I was packed off the see an alarmingly cheerful nurse, but perhaps it just seemed alarming because it was still early. She weighed me and didn't tell me the number (thank God!), took my blood pressure, and ran through yet more forms about family history and what blood tests they were going to order.

Blood test forms and random vitamin samples in hand, I was packed off back to the ultrasound room to try again. This time I didn't bother waiting for the doctor to leave the room before I took off my clothes. I just got to it. I figured she'd seen it all before anyway, and we were just wasting time with unnecessary modesty. So, I stripped and hopped back on the table.

It took one more go of me lying on my side before the baby cooperated and sat where she was supposed to. The doctor made the effort of pointing out all her body parts and even did a 3D picture (which looked totally weird and alien). She informed me that, in line with my own suspicions, I was 13 and a half weeks pregnant and would be due on the 12th of July. She told us to meet her at the reception to schedule the next appointment and she'd give us some pictures too.

As I wiped the blue goo off myself for the second time and got dressed I almost tripped getting into my trousers, causing my husband to say, "Don't fall and hurt my daughter." I retaliated with, "She's totally fine! The only person who'll get bruised is me." But I could tell from the look on his face he wasn't really scolding me. He was just excited to say the words, "my daughter."

We left the clinic to go next door for the blood tests. There was (unsurprisingly) more paperwork but I was seen pretty quickly. My husband asked if I wanted him to come in but I told him not to bother. It was only a blood test and I'm not afraid of needles. Don't get me wrong, I'm not fond of having my blood taken, but I've had enough blood tests over the years (and I used to give blood) that I know exactly what I'm in for.

I sat in the chair and the man asked me which arm I wanted it taken from. I told him, "Everyone always chooses the left and they always pick the same vein. You'll see it." I did actually once have a man say to me, "You have great veins," just before taking my blood. It was definitely one of the weirder compliments I've ever had.

I stared into my lap and clenched my right hand. I may have been poked with needles many times before, but that doesn't mean it doesn't hurt, nor does it mean I want to watch it. But as far as pain goes, it rates with a teeth clenching, not a screaming episode.

I didn't really know what tests they'd ordered (I'd just agreed to the iron work-up and whatever genetic ones they recommended) but there seemed to be a never-ending supply of phials he was filling up. No joke, there must have been at least eight. It was so many that towards the end my left hand started to feel a bit tingly and weird due to lack of circulation.

Just when I thought we were done he told me I had to give a urine sample too. I had already used the bathroom twice next door because your bladder is supposed to be empty for an ultrasound so they can see better, but one of the perks of being pregnant is that you pretty much always need the bathroom.

"How much do you need?" I asked, a bit unsure of what was left in the tank.

"If you get half a cup you're over-achieving, and that's great."

I managed the half a cup, plonked it in the pee sample in-tray and we left.

I emailed my parents and best friend to tell them it wasn't twins, and that I would be having a girl. Both my Mother and my best friend got back very excited about it. My Mother never chose to know the gender of her babies, but I agree with the doctor I saw, who said, "It helps you bond earlier if you know." It certainly feels more personal to call the baby "she" rather than "it."

My next appointment is in three weeks' time and until then I'm just going to keep doing what I'm doing. We may try and choose a baby name sooner rather than later. It shouldn't be too hard. All the girls on the English side of the family have names that begin with the letter J. So, I'll only have one letter to choose from, which certainly cuts the job down to size.

Chapter 17- Pregnancy Skin and Lack of Sex Drive

Okay, this has got to be right up there with morning sickness as one of the most unpleasant pregnancy side effects. Due to the fact that my hormones are going wacko, my skin has been complaining too. I used to have terrible skin as a teenager and young adult, and it's only really in the last year or two that it's improved due to me drastically changing my diet.

The reason I get so massively annoyed about bad skin is that a) I'm super pale so everything shows badly on my skin, and b) my skin seems to heal slowly. Meaning that when my skin is bad, it doesn't recover for weeks, sometimes months. Before I got pregnant I was finally beginning to enjoy almost clear skin. So, the abrupt downturn has been particularly distressing for me because I was so close to feeling confident enough to leave the house without make-up. And now I don't see that happening any time soon.

Apparently, according to Web MD, 1 in 2 women will suffer pregnancy acne due to the rising levels of progesterone in your body. Let me just say, THIS IS NOT COOL! Not only do I feel like a sick, beached whale, I now have to contend with bad skin that makes my self-esteem smaller than a gnat. I am not happy!

I'm in a guerrilla war with my daughter. You see, my body reacts very badly to certain foods. If I eat much sugar at all, I get spots. However, over the last month if I didn't eat at least natural sugar (think bananas, or in a pinch, a glass of coke), I felt nauseous. The first trimester, for me, has been a tug of war between my vanity and my desire to not throw up. For the most part, my desire to not throw up won, much to my skin's annoyance.

Finally, at 14.5 weeks pregnant, I seem to be able to go without sugar (like coke), and, at last, my skin is starting to clear up. It's really upsetting to have bad skin, especially when it's not just confined to your face. Mine affects my chest and back too. You don't want to go out, you never let people see you without make-up, you don't wear anything low cut, and you certainly don't wear a swimsuit.

It seems so unfair that on top of everything else, pregnant women have to deal with bad skin, especially because there are so few treatment options available for them. Like with most things, we're just expected to put up with it because, "It's good for the baby." Well fuck that! My husband won't be attracted to me if I look like a pizza, will he?

It got me thinking though, because the quality of your skin is a sign of internal health, and indigenous people don't seem to have the same skin issues that western cultures have. I have always felt there had to be a bigger link to my skin problems than simply "hormones." And over time, I did work out that most of my issues stem from food.

Now I'm not saying that all people will be as sensitive to foods as I am. I do believe I have autoimmune issues that make mine worse, but there are certain foods that are just big NO's for me. They include: grains of any form, sugar, and dairy (it gives me cystic acne – the worst type). There are others but I won't bore you with a big list. The problem is that pregnant women often either need or crave a lot of foods that can make your skin really bad.

I'm not saying I've found a way around the problem. I vowed not to eat crap when I fell pregnant but even I was reaching for the coke bottle in an effort to quell the nausea. All I can say is that no matter how much you crave it, once the nausea stops, cut your consumption of acne aggravating foods. Perhaps next time around I'll find a solution to this dilemma that doesn't involve sugar, but I haven't yet.

I was pretty staggered by the statistics too. 1 in 2 women will get pregnancy acne? That's massive! It certainly doesn't fit in line with the "glowing" pregnancy myth. People think, "Oh, pregnancy will be great. I'll be glowing and content. I'll do yoga and drink green juices. It'll be fabulous." In reality, we're crawling from the bed to hang over a toilet and shunning all food except the stuff that makes our skin crap. Hardly the fairytale version of events.

While we're on the subject of unfair things, where's my sex drive? I was told it would come back in the second trimester. I'm still waiting. It's like someone has turned the switch off. I'm just not interested, which is totally out of character. My husband and I used to have sex every day. Now it's more like every two or three days, and even then it's only because I comply, not really because I'm in the mood.

I don't know if it's somehow linked to the fact that I haven't been feeling very good about myself lately (what with the growing bump, massive tits, and bad skin), but I've just not really wanted to be that intimate. I know there'll be a lot of women out there saying, "So just don't have sex then!" But I don't really think that's fair on my husband. He still wants me, and it's not really that hard to spread my legs for 10-15 minutes. I'm just not enjoying it like I used to.

I feel remarkably detached at the moment, almost as though my lower half isn't hooked up to my brain anymore. I don't get that turned on and I don't seem to feel very much. It's very odd. But I suppose I should have expected it. The last time I tried the pill the same thing happened. My sex drive disappeared faster than food currently does in front of me. All I can say is that I hope it doesn't last long.

Whilst I understand there's no real reason for me to be interested in sex right now (I'm pregnant: mission accomplished!) I'm just bummed out! So far I've had every single damn pregnancy side effect bar this one. Let me repeat that: I've had EVERY negative side effect and the ONLY side effect I haven't had is the ONLY good one. Fuck you Mother Nature. You suck!

I suppose a lot of people are of the opinion that "it's just sex" and it's not that important. But I think it is. Certainly, it used to be to me, and I don't like the fact that I've changed my attitude to it so much since becoming pregnant. I'm not the only one bummed out either. My husband is a bit too. Sure, he's glad I've not told him we can't have sex, but I can tell he misses how enthusiastic I used to be about it. Luckily, he's mature enough to also know that this is temporary, and once I give birth and my hormones return to normal, things will go back to normal in that respect.

Maybe, in a few weeks when my skin has healed and I'm more into the second trimester, things will change. But right now, I'd say things are still pretty rubbish. I'm sure they'd improve massively with a martini (or at least, I'd care less about everything being crap), but I can't have one… yet.

I'm just dreading going through this again. I think you have to really, REALLY want children to be okay with all this, and I don't want them that much. If you include breastfeeding and potential post-natal depression, my baby is taking two or more years of my life. TWO OR MORE YEARS. I'm young enough that that seems like a really long time. I'm not sure I can bear to feel this crap for two years.

The only thing I can hope for is that my next child is a boy and the myth that pregnancy symptoms with girls' are worse is true, and that it won't be that bad the second time around, because at this point, I'm seriously doubting I'll want to do this more than once. I know everyone says you change your mind, but I'm not so convinced. The last time I got horrifically drunk I said I'd never do it again until the memory of the 4 day hangover faded from my mind. It's been over five years and I've still not forgotten it, and I've never gotten that drunk again. I'm wondering if this may end up being a similar thing.

There just seems to be so few people I can talk to about all this stuff. The moment you complain they just say, "It'll be worth it in the end." I guess they're trying to be supportive, but frankly that's not what I want to hear. I want someone to say, "I know. It's shit." but they don't. They just expect me to endure it like some sort of martyr because I'm so enamored with the miracle of creating life that I'm okay with putting up with all this crap.

I swear, if one more person says "it'll be worth it" I'm going to slap them. I just don't think they understand. Either they've never had kids, are men, or have had kids but seem to have forgotten about the horrors of pregnancy, or they had an easy pregnancy, so can't understand either. I actually read an article the other day about a bunch of men in a publishing house who spent a month wearing a pregnancy suit to see what later term pregnancy was actually like for women. The interview I read was ten days into the experiment and they were already admitting it was hell, and that wasn't even taking into account the trials of actually sustaining someone from your own body. All they had to do was carry around the weight.

I remember reading another study where a bunch of men volunteered to see what labor was really like on a pain level. Maybe they wanted to see whether women were justified in scoffing at their headaches as pathetic in comparison to what they have to go through. They had a bunch of electronic stimulant pads strapped to their stomach (a bit like those toning belts) and they cranked up the dial to full. Want to know how long some of them lasted? 40 minutes. After only half an hour to 40 minutes some were screaming and in such agony the experiment had to be stopped. And these are the sorts of people who say, it'll be worth it."

My husband has continually told me he expects me to swear bloody murder at him and blame him during birth. But I think unless he says something stupid like, "Just remember it's worth it!" then I won't lay into him. As far as I'm concerned right now, all this stuff IS NOT worth it. Maybe I'll change my mind, but I'm not going to belittle how appalling this is by justifying it away with the phrase 'it's worth it in the end."

Chapter 18- Weighty Issues, Vitamin Pushers, and Home Births

So, I had to go back to the doctors to meet the actual doctor this time. Only, unlike the nurse, she decided to tell me how much weight I'd gained since my last visit, three weeks ago. 11 pounds! She told me because apparently, that was "a little high." I tried to point out that my boobs had grown 3 cup sizes in 6 weeks and that food was not going through my system very fast, but she just said, "We'll keep an eye on it."

I was just really angry because I'm not great at math but I can do basic addition, and I don't want to know how much weight I gain during this. As far as I'm concerned, I'm only gaining what's necessary for the baby. I can still see my wrist bones, I can still see my collar bones and I can still see my cheekbones. I am not getting fat. I am just gaining weight on my stomach and boobs. And that's fine. I don't need anyone aggravating my body image issues by informing me of how much weight I'm putting on. There is a difference between fat and weight!

The next annoying thing that happened was that she tried to make me go on vitamin pills, like the nurse had in my last appointment. Now, I know that pregnant women have an increased need for iron and folic acid, but, ahem… I'm not eating any crap. There are a LOT of vegetables and meat in my everyday diet. I shouldn't, and don't, need vitamin pills.

However, despite my refusals, I did buy another bottle of pregnancy vitamins that claimed to be gentle on the stomach. I had refused to take the previous ones because they made me nauseous and I'd had more than enough of that, thank you very much. It turned out they were gentle on my stomach, but not the rest of my digestive system.

The problem is the vitamins in vitamin pills aren't that bioavailable, particularly the iron. Meaning they aren't very easily absorbed by the body. As a result, they constipated me for three days, and when I finally did manage to push one out it hurt so much I thought something had ripped. Needless to say, I stopped taking them immediately, and I will just be eating more red meat from now on.

News of my pregnancy is also slowly spreading among my husband's friends. The other day one of them was telling me how I should consider a home birth and do hypnotherapy to manage the pain. I almost wanted to spit out my drink. I am not one for "woo-woo" treatment. Hypnosis isn't as "hippy" a treatment as, say, homeopathy, but it's not one I'm willing to try for what will undoubtedly be the worst pain of my life.

Besides, I already know I'm not susceptible to hypnosis. We had a hypnotist come to my school once and he did a test on the crowd to determine the most susceptible people for his demonstration. I was not one of them. My mind is not easily swayed by outside influences. I like to make my own mind up on things.

At first I was totally against the notion of a home birth and I flatly told my husband I was not doing it, even though he was keen on the idea. But I've had time to think about it since and I can see some positives and negatives. On the plus side, assuming all goes well, I wouldn't have to stay in hospital overnight. I could just stay at home with my husband, where all my food and comfy bed is. On the negative side, if you need an epidural, it can only be done in a hospital.

So, now I'm torn. I would rather not have to be kept in hospital, but I don't know how bad the pain will be. I am a fairly gritty person and I can handle a pretty high level of pain. But the level of pain is at least, in part, going to be determined by how big my daughter is. There is a big difference between pushing out something that is six pounds versus ten. A BIG difference.

I know that Miranda Kerr gave birth to her ten-pound son without an epidural, but even she has admitted in interviews that it was "a challenge" (to put it mildly). I'm not sure I'd be up for that "challenge" myself. I'm not quite as zen as she is. I'm a bit too worried that something might rip down there, and then I'd definitely want to be high as a kite if that happens. There either needs to be an epidural on hand or a bottle of gin, because if it gets too bad, I'm going to need one or the other.

The other thing that's putting me off from a home birth is the fact that we live in a semi-detached house with fairly lame soundproofing. I'm not sure I want the neighbors (and the entire street for that matter) to hear me screaming. I don't really want an audience, even if they are just an audible one. I don't want any more people than necessary there to witness the birth, because lord knows I'm going to look terrible and it'll probably sound like someone is being murdered in the house.

I'm pretty scared of giving birth. While I am looking forward to having my daughter out so she can start living off her own reserves and give my body a break, it hasn't lessened my fear of actually giving birth. One of the reasons human births are so traumatic is because we have such big brains. Other animals can give birth to babies that are vastly more developed than ours. You see them plop out and half an hour later they're walking. But due to the huge size of the human baby's brain, birth is difficult and we expel babies than can't do anything for themselves but scream, eat, and poop.

My mother and sister have threatened to come over for the birth, but I'm not sure how wise that is. My sister isn't really a baby person either, and my mum and I will likely come close to killing each other due to exhaustion and wacko hormones. I know everyone says it's great to have help but it may be a bit like learning to drive, in that they recommend you don't learn from your family. My husband has been teaching me to drive and we've not come anywhere close to a divorce, so we may be alright on our own.

Someone at a party recently told me I had to get my daughter on the waiting list for day care now because there are huge queues, but I'm not really sure she needs to be on the waiting list. I mean, I work from home. I'll be looking after her. I don't want my daughter to effectively be raised by other people. My mother worked for a while in a nursery and she told me some of the kids came to view it as their home because they were there from eight in the morning until six at night, and barely saw their parents. I don't really intend for my children to spend too much time in daycare, maybe a few afternoons or mornings a week when they're 2 or 3 to learn some social skills with other kids, but no more than that. I'll get a proper break when they start school.

Later at the party people started telling me what middle name I should give my daughter. Now, I'm not sure if people feel they have the right to tell me what to name my daughter because they have kids and therefore deem themselves experienced, or because the wine was talking and they lacked the normal manners to keep their opinions on MY daughter's names to themselves (probably the latter), but I didn't really appreciate the forcefulness of it. Needless to say, I bailed on the party shortly afterwards. I don't want to be seen as a party pooper, but parties aren't that fun when everyone is four glasses of wine in and you're stone cold sober. So, I retired to my bedroom to watch Netflix in my pyjamas in peace.

Chapter 19– Baby Movements, Nipple Hell, and Sneezing Fits

I was informed that I might start to feel baby movements as early as 18 weeks but I don't think I really felt much until about 19 weeks, and even then, it wasn't a particularly profound moment. I had read online about all these women who had been overjoyed at feeling the first "flutter" of movement from their baby but when I felt it all I thought was, "Huh! Feels like gas." Not particularly poetic.

I have now graduated from the gas-like gurgling to actual recognizable movement. But actually, it's a bit annoying. The other day I was shattered and doing my level best to lie down and take a nap when my daughter decided that that was the opportune moment to try out some gymnastic moves. I ended up shouting, "Knock it off! I'm trying to sleep here!" to my own stomach. I have morphed into the crazy mom talking to her unborn child.

I'm still waiting for my husband to feel any movement. The other day he asked why I could feel it with my hand but he never did. I pointed out that he's far more interested in checking out my boobs than my stomach, and even when he does have his hand in the right place to feel anything (when he's the big spoon at bedtime), he falls asleep before anything happens.

My husband is one of those people who falls asleep at the drop of a hat. I greatly envy him that gift. I do sleep better now that I have completely cut caffeine out of my life, but still nowhere near as well as he does. He's like a child. You count to ten and he's out cold. And he can sleep anywhere. He once took a nap in a tree.

I wasn't always a troubled sleeper. As a child, I once fell asleep in my dinner, much to my parents' amusement. My brain registered full and I went face first into a plate of spaghetti with a snore. My brother almost did the same at a restaurant, but we tied him upright to the chair with my Mother's scarf, thereby avoiding another face-dinner situation.

This may be wishful thinking but I suspect that between my husband and me we may actually be able to cope with the broken nights of a newborn. My nights have been broken for as long as I can remember, so getting up several times a night isn't going to be anything new to me, and my husband has no trouble taking naps during the day and falling straight back to sleep at night. So, fingers crossed, we might actually be able to cope.

I know my husband will eventually feel the baby move, but I suspect I'll get a response similar to the one I got at the first ultrasound and when I told him I was pregnant: a polite but fairly unemotional response. He's the sort of person who doesn't really acknowledge something until it's right in front of his face. So he probably won't get emotional and excited until his daughter is LITERALLY in front on him (apparently my growing stomach isn't evidence enough – I have to pop the baby out before he'll take notice).

I have another ultrasound this week so I'll get a good idea of just how much wriggling is going on then. It's apparently one of the more important ultrasounds and is going to last 45 minutes. I'm not really sure what they're going to be looking at for 45 minutes, I mean, my daughter isn't that big yet, but I guess I'll find out. Hopefully no one will try and fob more vitamin pills off on me.

The other day, after a crying fit (hey, sometimes the size of my mountainous boobs just gets me down) my husband made the mistake of saying "things will get better." Little did he know that earlier that day I had stupidly researched all the things that would be in store for me between now and giving birth. I looked at him somewhat confused and said, "No, nothing's going to get better."

Granted, I don't feel sick and I don't have headaches anymore, but, back to my boobs, my nipples feel like someone's trying to cut them off when I get cold. I'm serious! The pain is agonizing and the only thing I can do to lessen it is have a hot shower or sit in front of a heater. Nothing else helps. So, despite the fact that I live 5 minutes from a pool, I can't go swimming because after 10 lengths my nipples are simply KILLING ME!

What's more, I have developed the worst allergies ever. In fact, my nose seems bigger due to the swelling from constantly sneezing (and I don't just mean once or twice, we're talking seven to ten times in a row here) and blowing my nose. Occasionally, my husband puts some tissue in front of me when I'm sniffing as a gentle hint to blow my nose, but it's POINTLESS. No matter how much I blow my nose I'm still bunged up.

Oh, and while we're on the subject of sneezing, thanks to my daughter flooding my body with hormones to make all my muscles relax to accommodate her, sometimes when I sneeze now I end up wetting my pants a bit (usually on the 7th or 8th sneeze). It's both humiliating and annoying. The only solution I've found is to cross my legs whenever I can feel a sneeze coming. It's far from practical, but at least it stops me having to do so much damn laundry.

But my spell of dry panties will be short lived. Soon my daughter will be big enough to kick my bladder and force me to wet myself again. MORTIFICADO! I mean, I'm 27 years old and before I got pregnant ALL my muscle control was perfectly good. I didn't have a weak pelvic floor at all, but now I feel like I'm in my eighties and need a diaper. At least we have self-service check-out machines these days so I won't have to look at the cashier when I inevitably buy incontinence pads.

I did used to wonder why there were so many incontinence pads in supermarkets. A few times I would think, "Surely there can't be that many incontinent people out there?" but now I know. It's mostly for pregnant woman. That's why they put them down the aisle with the tampons and pregnancy tests. It had never occurred to me before. But now I know. It's the one stop shop aisle for Mother Nature hell.

One of the laughable things women often say to me about pregnancy is, "Oh, it must be so nice to not have your period every month." Ignoring the fact that I've felt too crappy to even really notice I've not had to deal with a period, I will soon have to wear pads again. But this time, not just for a week each month; every sodding day, because I won't be able to predict when my daughter will want to play football with my bladder. And that's not even getting started on when she'll be able to kick my cervix and send me buckling to my knees in pain.

And let's talk about skin again, not only is it massively unfair that pregnant women have to contend with teenage skin again, once your flare ups are over, your skin just doesn't fucking heal for like, forever! I'm not sure whether it's just because my body is too busy being concerned about making someone else, or whether it's to do with my immune system being down, but it is taking my skin WEEKS to heal from even a simple scratch. I burnt my wrist on the oven making croissants for Christmas and it's taken TWO MONTHS to heal properly. I don't know what to do other than drink more water and try to get more nutrients in my diet.

On the subject of healing, not only will I pretty much guaranteed poop during birth (how glamorous, I'm going to poop in front of a room full of people – now my husband is definitely not allowed below the waist during the birth), I may also tear "down there" from the task of forcing something so big out of something so small. Meaning they'll have to stitch me up. How horrifying!

Whilst, from what I can tell, women heal just fine from their stitches, it apparently makes peeing for the next while a torturous experience, never mind sex (which is on most men's minds after about, oh, 24 hours). And it's not game over once the baby is out. No Sir. Next comes the "afterbirth", where you expel the placenta. To be honest, it's sounding more and more like my body is going to be doing its very best to completely toss out the contents of everything inside me. They really ought to just film birth and release it as a horror movie. I'm sure it's more horrifying than anything that's come out of Hollywood recently. It'd probably win an award.

So, you can see why when my husband said, "It'll get better" I quite simply didn't believe him. The only thing that seems to be doing well at all is my hair and nails, which seem to be growing at an incredible rate, but even that's a double edged sword as I'm told lots of my hair will fall out after I give birth and my nails will go back to their previous state of bending rather than breaking. Seriously, how does anyone do this more than once? They should give out medals.

Chapter 20- Vaginal Jacking, Balloon Boobs, Backache, and Hot Tub Bans

I had my anatomy ultrasound the other day and apparently everything is fine, not that I'd know. Most of the stuff on the ultrasound just looks like a blob to me. I undressed as soon as the technician showed us in and hopped on the table because, frankly, modesty wastes time and so much of my modesty has already been ripped out from underneath me due to being pregnant that I saw little point in pretending I still had any.

The technician went through and checked out all my daughter's body parts but all I could make out was the head and spine. The rest was a bit of a blur, but she sped through going, "This is the right hand and this the left foot." I just felt like I was in one of those shrink offices where someone was showing me ink splodges and making up a description of what it looked like while I politely nodded.

We got more ultrasound pictures but they look a lot like the first set we got (and basically like every ultrasound picture I've ever seen of every baby ever, regardless of whose it was). Then I was told I had to see the doctor again. So I followed another nurse, who weighed me (I didn't look), took my blood pressure, and told me I'd be having a full exam with pap test, cervical sample… the works. She handed me a pink gown, told me to undress and to leave the opening at the front.

I sat for what must have been twenty minutes in my flimsy pink gown, really wishing I could put my bra back on (seriously, at this size I need some structural support). It was taking so long that my husband disappeared and re-appeared with snacks before the doctor arrived. He then proceeded to sit and watch my breast exam with his snacks as though he was at the cinema. It only got truly weird when the doctor proceeded to get the speculum out and jack me open as my husband munched his bag of revels and idly chatted to the doctor about their upcoming office move.

Afterwards, my husband asked me if it had hurt because I had been pulling some funny faces. I told him half of it was that it's just not that fun to have something cold and metal put inside you, and the other half is that no one enjoys having their insides pried open and skin torn out (apparently he didn't know what a pap test actually consisted of – he does now!).

Thankfully, the doctor didn't tell me how much weight I'd gained since I last saw her. She just said my weight gain was "back on track", whatever that meant. I remarked that I would have been alarmed if my boobs had gained another two cup sizes in a month, but she just casually told me they weren't done growing and would get even bigger.

I left feeling decidedly depressed about the news for my boobs. They're already ridiculous, so the news that they were going to get even bigger was pretty upsetting. I'm already in porn star territory with regard to size. The only place left to go is Japanese anime porn territory (think watermelons). I'm not looking forward to it. Every time I look at my boobs in the mirror I hate what I see, but unlike my stomach after giving birth, they won't decrease in size until I stop breastfeeding. So, I've a good while to go before they deflate to a more manageable size.

Furthermore, bras in large sizes are absurdly expensive in the U.S. It's just not fair. They're taking advantage of the fact that busty gals CAN'T do without a good bra by charging us an arm and a leg for them. Bigger bras were a lot easier to get a hold of in the UK. Marks and Spencer did great bras up to a GG for around 25 pounds. Really good value, and they probably had bigger sizes too, I just never looked because I never needed to. The bras I bought a month ago are seriously snug (and they're a 32 GG – which in the U.S. is an H!) and I'm even busting out of my stretchy sports bra.

My bra prospects are particularly alarming because if my boobs get much bigger I'm going to run out of letters of the alphabet. I think most bras stop at a J or a K, and I'm not that far off that now. Furthermore, I'm almost finding it impossible to find a good maternity bra in a large size because, let's face it, at my size you need structural engineering, and most maternity bras are wireless. I mean, WTF? They claim it's for comfort but there is just NO way a bra can support you at that size without wires.

I happen to know wireless maternity bras suck for large busts for a fact because I bought some, and they're crap. The fabric on the band just kind of folds over and doesn't support the weight of my boobs properly. Most of the weight of your boobs is supposed to be supported by the band on a bra that goes around your ribcage, not by the shoulder straps. But these bras, because the band doesn't sit properly on my ribcage (because my boobs are too massive) they don't support my boobs. So all the weight is going on my shoulders and the cups sag down over the bra band in a really unflattering fashion because the straps simply CANNOT support such weight.

While I'm on the subject of boobs, there is SO much pressure to breastfeed. I know it's best for the baby, but at some point I'm going to get REALLY fed up of having massive hooters that leak on my t-shirts and I'll want to stop, but there doesn't seem to be any real consensus on when you should stop. Some women only last a few weeks, whereas others do it for years. I reckon I'll try and do it for the first six months and then see how fed up I am. By that point my daughter should be able to eat "solid" foods and so the demand for me to provide all sustenance will reduce.

Another drawback to my truly ginormous hooters is back pain. I was told back pain wouldn't be an issue until the later months of pregnancy, but they'd clearly not factored in the two melons I'd have to carry along with my bundle of joy. Needless to say, my back is not happy and it is telling me about it, loudly.

I read that sleeping on your back can make things worse so I've tried sleeping on my side, but I just wake up on my back. I don't know how to stop that. I've tried sitting up straighter, stretching more, and wearing proper fitting bras, but everything only provides temporary relief. It hurts when I've been standing or walking for more than 30 minutes. It hurts when I try and get out of bed, which I do several times a night because I have to get up to pee. It hurts when I'm merely sitting at my desk, writing. The only thing that has helped is going to the hot tub at the swimming pool, but as I found out today, I'm not supposed to do that.

According to various people, I'm not allowed to get in a hot tub for more than 10 minutes because it can cause my body temperature to rise and that's dangerous for the baby. I just wanted to cry when I found that out. The ONLY thing that's stopping my back from aching like I've been carrying a hippo for a fortnight, I'm not allowed to do.

Now I know you'll all be saying, "So just get in the regular pool!" but as I explained earlier, I can't, because NIPPLE HELL! My nipples absolutely KILL me when I'm cold. Unless the temperature outside is scorching (which it's not in March) I simply cannot sit in cold water, or even swim in it for long at all. Even cold air can set them off. So, I'm now left with no feasible options to reduce the strain on my back. It doesn't seem to matter which way I lie, it all hurts.

I feel as though my daughter has morphed into the fun police. Due to her, I can't drink, smoke (not that I do anyway), take most painkillers or allergy medicine to stop my nose from turning into a tap, take laxatives to un-cork my digestive track, or take medication to help me sleep through my aches and pains (and her kicking). And now I can't go in the hot tub. THIS SUCKS BALLS!

My aches and pains got so bad the other day that I could barely walk. Apparently, the ligaments on the right side of my stomach weren't too happy about trying to accommodate a football, and went on strike. It felt like I was being stabbed, repeatedly, for TWO DAYS! I would either end up whimpering or literally yelping involuntarily when I tried to get up, move in bed, and get in and out of the car... everything I did hurt. I was limping around the house barely able to stand on my right foot, to the point where it was looking like I'd need a walking stick if it didn't stop soon. Thankfully, it only lasted two days but I have the feeling I'm not out of the woods yet. It could strike again at any moment.

My husband and I have taken some measures to try and reduce my back pain. I decided the other day that it was time to put my handbag away and switch to a backpack. Unfashionable though it is, it does do wonders for my lower back pain. One of the reasons pregnant women get lower back pain is because our center of gravity has shifted due to us carrying so much weight on our front. But when I put the shopping in my backpack and walked home, all of a sudden I was balanced again, and by the time I got home, my lower back pain had practically disappeared. I may just fill the backpack with rocks and carry it around all the time because, lord knows, no over the counter painkillers have done anything for me.

We have also purchased a "body pillow" which looks more like a donut than a pillow. It got five stars on Amazon from reviewers (most of whom were pregnant though a few husbands admitted to trying it) so my husband ordered one. I was fairly dubious of it at first because there are some downsides. It takes up a huge amount of the bed and it puts a rather firm barrier between me and my husband. Whilst my husband can sleep just fine snuggled up against me I often can't sleep unless I'm spread out, so this ought to be a good thing, except I do like being hugged, especially when I'm feeling crappy (which is a lot of the time now).

My experience with the body pillow is that it helps me sleep better providing nothing else is actually wrong. If I have sore muscles, restless legs, or I feel unwell, it doesn't improve anything (whereas a hug does, at least from a morale standpoint). But if everything else is okay, I do sleep better because it forces me to stay on my side more, it lifts my knees to be in line with my spine, and there's a bit I can wedge between my boobs to separate them (sweaty boobs stuck together isn't pleasant).

However, despite the body pillow's many positives, I am still faced with the slight dilemma of where to put my arm. In the diagram the woman looks like her arm is just crooked with her hand under the pillow, but I can't do that. I can't have my boobs resting on my bicep because they're so heavy that they cut off the circulation to my lower arm, and there are few things more alarming than waking up thinking there's a stranger in the bed because you don't recognize your own arm.

Sigh. My woe related boob saga goes on. Stay tuned for further updates.

Chapter 21– Arm Pain, Hugs from Random Children, and Unwelcome Jokes

So we're back from a weekend conference. We stayed in a pretty nice hotel with a pool and the room had a mini kitchen so I could cook for myself. Normally, I love hotels because the air con is awesome, the beds are comfy, and the curtains block out all the light (meaning I can sleep in more) but I didn't sleep that well. I don't know if it was because it was a strange bed, because I didn't have my body pillow, because my husband didn't return from the conference until 10 or 11 at night, or whether it was because I was a bit under the weather, but by the end of the three days I was pretty shattered and just wanted to go home.

However, the pool at the hotel was awesome! I think perhaps it was because we were further inland so the air temperature was hotter, and so at about 2pm it was hot enough outside (and the pool was warm enough inside) that I could happily float about for half an hour without my nipples complaining. It was bliss, even more so because the pool was so beautifully twinkly and sparkly in the sunlight. How can that not put you in a good mood?

There was also a bath in the hotel bathroom, which I thoroughly enjoyed. At home we just have a shower unit in our bathroom but I still sit down in it (I get tired. Don't judge me). I used to love taking long baths and would often read in them for an hour, just soaking in the hot water, and it was great to be able to do that again. Although I confess, this time I didn't read. I watched *The Great British Bake Off* on my phone because I've always felt you can't possibly be in a bad mood when there's Mary Berry and cake.

However, as great as baths are, there was a major problem. You see, my stomach muscles are somewhat compromised at the moment, meaning sitting up is a real struggle. Every time I tried to sit up in the bath I could see them, stretched out over my stomach, straining to lift me up. I'm not THAT heavy, but they just don't seem to work the same way they used to. It's the same when I try and get out of bed. I'm not sure whether it's because my muscles are stretched so tight over my stomach, or whether it's due to the hormones causing my muscles to relax, but I now have to use my arms to haul myself upright or turn over if I'm lying down.

Usually, hotel baths have a rail on the wall for any disabled, old, pregnant, or weak people to pull themselves upright, and this hotel did… but it was on the wall with the shower unit, not on the wall next to where my head was in the bathtub. I suppose it was for caffeine deprived people to hold onto when standing in the shower early in the morning, but really, I think placing it on the wall closest to my head would have been better. That way I wouldn't have looked like an upturned turtle trying to right itself every time I wanted to get up to reach the soap, shampoo, conditioner, razor etc.

The downside of having to use my arms to haul myself around is that I seem to have developed bad pain in my left forearm. And when I say "bad" I'm being rather modest. Since we got back home it's been hurting so much that I've been unable to sleep. Painkillers are doing nothing but taking the edge off, and muscle rubs (such as Deep Heat or Ben Gay) are doing fuck all. I don't really know what to do about it except try not to use that arm and hope it goes away. I can't take any ibuprofen for muscle aches because YOU CAN'T TAKE THAT WHEN YOU'RE PREGNANT so I've taken to wearing a fluffy leg warmer (bring back the 80s!) on my arm in an effort to keep it warm and hopefully speed up recovery.

My husband was feeling sorry enough for me as we were leaving the hotel that he stopped in the middle of the corridor to give me a hug, which was perfectly fine as I'm not averse to a bit of PDA (public displays of affection), but there was a mother and her little girl walking past us at the time and the little girl decided she wanted in on the action. That's right. I got hugged by a stranger's child who then rather determinedly decided she wanted to hold my hand as we walked down the corridor.

Luckily, the mother was pretty chilled out about it and when my husband said we were going to have a girl too the little girl proceeded to pat my stomach. It's official. I've had my first non-family member pat my tummy. Normally I'd find it completely weird to have a stranger patting my stomach. I mean, in what other circumstance is it appropriate to pat a stranger? You don't pat someone's head when they say they have a headache. However, seeing as the little girl was about five years old and quite adorable, I didn't mind. I was just slightly baffled as to why she would want to get so close to someone she didn't know. The only conclusion I can think of is that I'm not scary anymore.

My father told me once about how he knew he'd turned a corner in his life when pretty, young women started sitting next to him on the train because in comparison to the other men in the carriage he was the "safe" choice. They'd take one look around, and decide to sit next to the businessman with the briefcase and umbrella rather than any man their age. I feel I'm turning a similar corner, where I seem to be emitting some sort of maternal vibe that acts as a homing beacon to children.

I've always been good with kids, and I like kids, but I've not generally been someone who looked that approachable on the street. Certainly, in London people rarely spoke to me on the street and my sister used to liken me to a velociraptor when I was walking about with a purpose. I know it's arguable that part of the reason I'm more approachable now is that I don't live in a city anymore so my aggression levels have naturally decreased (public transport in rush hour, and the London Underground in particular, makes you angry), but I've been away from the city for a year and a half now and I've not had random children try to hug me, so I reckon something else is at play here.

Another thing that's adding to my sleep woes is the fact that my baby's wriggling is getting a lot more noticeable, but it really seemed to get out of control when we stopped at the cinema on the way back from the hotel. I wanted to see Cinderella because, you know, it's a fairy tale and I could do with something a little more pleasant than reality right now, but we ended up seeing American Sniper because that's what my husband wanted to see (next time it will be Cinderella – I need to see those Swarovski shoes!).

American Sniper is a good film but what I had failed to take into account when I agreed to see it was the noise level. In my opinion, cinemas are too loud in general, regardless of what film you choose to watch, but because most of this film was set in a war zone it rather exacerbated the problem. Whilst I could just cover my ears during the loud parts, the same could not be said for my baby. Apparently, even unborn babies don't like loud noises, because she would squirm and kick whenever there was gunfire (which was most of the film). I ended up placing both mine and my husband's jackets over my stomach in an attempt to muffle the noise and make her stop.

Avoiding the cinema is just another thing to add to the list of things I can't do because of the baby. I swear the list gets longer by the day, and, at 23 weeks, I'm starting to get fed up. I'm fed up of violently sneezing ten times in a row multiple times a day where any sneeze could result in me having to change my underpants (top tip: always carry spares), I'm fed up of watching other people drink and eat things I can't at parties (seriously, I never cared much for shellfish before but now I really want it), I'm fed up of my boobs making my life hell, I'm fed up of everything hurting all the time, I'm fed up of getting sick so often, and I'm fed up of people making pregnancy jokes to me.

That last one is particularly getting to me at the moment. In other circumstances people usually wait to make jokes about your misfortune until whatever you're going through is over. Otherwise you risk the "too soon" situation. However, this rule seems to have gone out of the window with regard to pregnancy because people seem to think it's okay to make jokes about it all the time, even my husband, who has recently taken to joking about my size by calling me "rotund" or "tubby." I know he's joking (because you'd only know I'm pregnant by looking at my stomach and boobs. The rest of my body doesn't seem to have changed much), but as someone who has suffered plenty of body image issues, it's not great. If he continues, he'll get slapped at some point.

Similarly, other people, especially those who have kids, make lots of jokes about "You're pregnant? What were you thinking?" It's like, "Well, gee thanks but I can't fucking bail out of it now!" I'm already miserable, don't go on and tell me how miserable I'll be once my baby is born. I'm already dreading birth enough that I don't need to start feeling shitty about what's going to happen afterwards.

I would have thought that people who've had kids would know better, but they seem to have forgotten how traumatic this part is, and how much joking about a situation that is happening to me RIGHT NOW is insensitive. I particularly dislike how my husband laughs along to these jokes because (perhaps unreasonably) I feel they're laughing at me rather than with me. They're all having a good giggle at my situation while I'm standing in the corner, the one who is actually going through it, not feeling that any of it is particularly funny at all. As far as I'm concerned, people who make "you're in trouble now" jokes are as bad as people who say, "It'll be worth it in the end." They can all sod off.

But don't get me wrong. I'm not trying to start a pregnancy related gender war against my husband and all other men that joke about pregnant women. I know they can never fully understand what I'm going through, and I'd never wish this on them. I try really hard not going to snap and say stuff like, "You're headache is irrelevant. You try putting up with X, Y, Z for 9 months!" But I do wish they'd be a bit more understanding. I just need someone to listen when I feel down, to help me up off the floor when I'm stuck rather than laugh at me, and to give me more cuddles instead of making jokes about how spherical I'm getting. Pregnancy is a lonely venture. The last thing you need is people belittling your suffering by making you the butt of all jokes (especially if your butt has become massive!).

Chapter 22- Pregnancy Horror Stories
and Involuntary Diets

Something odd is happening. I'm losing interest in food. Maybe I'm just tired, but I'm not excited by meals anymore. If anything, they're proving a bit of a challenge because I don't seem to be able to eat very much in one go anymore. I find myself getting quite stuffed quite quickly but seeing as most of the foods I eat aren't that high in calories, I have to eat pretty frequently to stop from feeling like I have morning sickness again. It's a double-edged sword. Eat too much and I feel sick because there's no space in my stomach. Eat too little and I feel sick because my blood sugar goes too low. The solution just seems to be to try and eat all day, grazing, like a cow.

What's really funny is that while I'm not really that enamored with my dinner anymore, I'm obsessed with cooking programs. I love watching Nigella Lawson, and pretty much any baking program. But actually eating food, as opposed to watching it, is beginning to feel a bit like a chore. I'm eating slower than ever and have suddenly had involuntary portion restrictions imposed on me. A plate of food I could devour in 15 minutes is now a challenge and I'm so stuffed afterwards I can't touch anything else for a few hours.

But the prognosis for improvement isn't good. My internal organs are only going to get more squished from here on out. So my food intake is likely to continue to reduce until I'm eating child-like portions. But hey, maybe it'll make losing baby weight easier if my stomach's shrunk. Mind you, that's not taking into account how ravenously hungry I'll apparently be when I breastfeed.

The other day we had lunch with someone and they decided that halfway through my salad was the opportune moment to tell me a horror story about their wife giving birth. Now, given the spirit of this book, I don't mind people being honest about how tough it is. I expect it to be the worst thing I've ever gone through. What I do mind is people saying, "Afterwards she tried to stand up to go to the bathroom and collapsed. I thought she'd died. She'd lost so much blood."

Um… No! Not okay. Don't tell me that over lunch. I mean, firstly, I'm eating so not cool. Secondly, let's not mention the word death. You can tell me (preferably after lunch) about how long the labor was, how hard it was, how huge the baby was, that something went wrong, but let's just leave the notion of death out of it so we don't scare the first-time mom shitless. It's already terrifying. I don't need to start worrying that I might die too.

Maternal death rates in developed countries are pretty low but they do still happen. However, it's not something I want to dwell on, because, well, I don't have any choice but to give birth now. This is, in fact, one of the reasons I've avoided going to prenatal groups or having a baby shower. People seem to think it's okay to scare the shit out of mom's-to-be by telling them stories about every birth they know that went wrong. Every time someone starts one of these stories I just want to cry, "Please let me be ignorant for at least one birth!"

We had dinner out with a couple the other day whose children are practically grown up and they too jumped in on the "let's scare the pregnant woman" game. I didn't really know them very well, so I was trying to be polite by not telling them to shut the hell up, but when we got home I was so terrified I burst into tears and it took my husband half an hour and many cuddles to calm me down.

To try and take some of the fear factor away my husband bought me a book about pregnancy and birth but until recently I'd been too scared to open it. I knew I'd deal with it in my own time, and I did. The other weekend I opened it and read it from cover to cover, and contrary to everything I've said before, I came away convinced that I didn't want to have a hospital birth, certainly not in America.

I know earlier in this book I made my feelings on how I wanted to give birth perfectly clear: drug me up and maybe do a c-section. But I've changed my mind. The more I read of the book, the more convinced I became that the fewer interventions I had, the better. After all, if our bodies weren't designed to have children, then surely we'd have another way of reproducing?

I think my main fear is how much it will hurt. I've never had children and everyone tells me it'll be the worst pain I will have ever experienced. Now, from a psychological point of view, if you go into something convinced it will hurt like hell… it will hurt like hell. Anyone who disagrees with me hasn't heard of the placebo effect. Your brain can do wonderful things when it wants to. If you think something you've taken will lessen your pain, even if it's nothing but a sugar pill, you will feel less pain.

Furthermore, from what I read the U.S. is super trigger happy when it comes to artificially inducing labor if you go over your due date or if you don't progress fast enough once you get to the hospital (labor can stall). The problem with this is that these inducement drugs make contractions stronger (i.e. more painful). And once you start with the interventions, they just seem to carry on. They induce you, give you an epidural, cut you so your vagina opening is wider, and if you still take too long to pop the kid out, they suck it out with a vacuum, pull it out with some forceps, or decide an emergency C section is necessary.

I can't even begin to go into all the things that are wrong with this method of childbirth. Just take my advice, when you are ready, read Ina May's *Guide to Childbirth*. I'll confess I've stuck post-it notes over the photos of women giving birth (I have limits of what I want to see and squished slimy babies being squashed out of women's nether regions WAY oversteps the line), but she'll open your eyes to the risks no one tells you about in giving birth in the hospital.

It's funny that you only tend to hear horror stories about women who refused an epidural, or who chose to do a home birth. No one tells you about things that went wrong when people did everything the doctors and society expects of them. For example, everyone glosses over the fact that an epidural can leave you in pain for weeks, or that if it goes wrong it can leave you incontinent (my best friend knows someone who had that happen to them for 18 months after giving birth), or that if your body doesn't expel the placenta fast enough the doctors pull on it to try and get it out, which can make the bleeding worse.

Basically, plenty goes wrong in the hospitals, but no one seems to want to talk about those incidences. They only want to scare people who try and do anything different. I'm now set on a home birth because I know that way nothing will be done to me unless totally necessary. No one is going to induce me or cut me to hurry things along because they want their tea break. I will have endured my baby for nine sodding months by the time birth comes around. The least anyone else can do is be patient for a few extra hours while I get her out.

One of the added benefits of a home birth is that if labor lasts ages I can eat and drink. They don't let you do that in the hospital, just in case they have to do an emergency c-section. I also don't have to panic about when the right time is to go to the hospital. I won't be going anywhere. The midwife will come to me. I'll be following Ina May's advice, sitting down and doing my best to relax. I've already informed the husband that if I start to freak out I'm going to watch re-runs of *The Great British Bake Off* because nothing can go wrong when Mary Berry is talking. Nothing.

Chapter 23– Baby Crap, Inside Out Belly Buttons, and Disappearing Bikini Lines

I've reached the 6-month mark and we've started to think about what baby crap we'll need after my daughter is born. I know a lot of people get much of their baby stuff from a baby shower but I just don't see the point in me or anyone buying much new stuff these days. Babies outgrow everything (or throw up on it, poo on it, etc.) so fast that there's little point getting them new things.

We sent an email out to the university mailing list asking if anyone had any old baby stuff they didn't want anymore. So far, we have a basinet, a changing mat, a highchair and some clothes. We have outstanding offers for a car seat, a baby bath, a crib, a playpen, and a pushchair. Some of the people we have spoken to have just been like, "Thank God! I've been dying to get that stuff out of my garage for ages!"

I know a lot of new mums like to pour over baby clothes in the stores and get cute little matching outfits, but really, why bother? They'll outgrow everything before you have a chance to enjoy how cute they look because you'll be too tired or busy to really care about dressing them up. My brother barely got any new clothes until he was in his teens. He just got hand-me-downs from other boys on the street, and it was fine.

Of course, there are a few things you probably should buy new, like bottles and dummies (if you choose to use them – I don't really plan on it because it's such a hassle to sterilize everything). But for the most part, you don't need to get new things. Babies are expensive enough. There's no point making them more costly by dressing them up in baby Gucci. Save your money and by yourself a spa day. You'll freaking deserve one after all you've been through!

I'm not really that into pampering, and to be honest, it's getting harder and harder to do the minimal pampering that I do bother with. For example, my stomach has now overtaken my boobs in girth (this is quite an achievement) and it's proving extremely challenging to do my bikini line because, well, I can't really see it anymore. Even if I try to squash my tummy out of the way, I only get glimpses of it at best. Soon I'll have to resort to a mirror, but that could go disastrously wrong as everything will be back to front in the reflection.

Similarly, I used to paint my toenails, but it's getting more and more difficult to reach my toes. Even just shaving my legs is proving to be a challenge and I sit down to do it so I don't topple over in the shower. Even matters as simple as trying to get a suntan are a logistical nightmare. I can sunbathe my front, no problem, but I'm not able to lie on my stomach… so how do I suntan my back and the back of my legs? It's impossible to do on the pool loungers and the only solution I have found is to go to the beach, dig a hole in the sand and plonk my stomach in it.

Speaking of my stomach, have you ever wondered what the inside of your belly button looks like? Well, I hadn't until I realized I could literally turn mine inside out and have a look. That's right, the skin on my stomach is so stretched that if I press either side of my belly button I can literally turn it inside out (in case you didn't guess, I have an inny). It's both gross and funny. If you ever felt like cleaning out belly button fluff, this would be a good opportunity.

What I'm really amazed by is the fact I haven't gotten any stretch marks yet. I've gotten a few varicose veins, but no stretch marks, and It might have something to do with my avocado problem. I say "problem" because I have a problem showing any self-control around them. I can quite easily eat four in a day (I don't do this every day, but often enough to class it as a problem). However, I'm not in a rush to curb this habit because I read somewhere limiting your intake of good fats isn't good for your skin and seeing as I don't have any stretch marks yet, I'm not going to change something that might be working.

As the days drag by I'm beginning to feel more and more unwieldy. Luckily, instead of laughing at me when I try to get up or turn over, my husband now does his best to help me. He acknowledges how much I'm suffering (hard to miss at this point), which is probably why I didn't know until a month ago that'd he'd like three children. He's carefully kept his mouth shut about that for a long time and when I found out I was like, "What? Since when?!"

Apparently, my husband has always wanted three kids. It might be because he was an only child himself, or it could be that he wants a number greater than two to replace ourselves (nerd logic), but either way, it was news to me. As someone who was beginning to question whether she could even manage two, three seemed like an unlikely venture. I think it'll all depend on how the next one goes. If it's another nightmare pregnancy, it's game over.

I hadn't planned on having more than two kids because to be perfectly honest, I want my body and life back. Selfish? Absolutely! But why shouldn't I be? It's my life. Who says I have to spend years being an incubator? I don't like having other people live off my body supplies. Currently, my plan is to have this kid and then get the next kid in the oven pronto. By those calculations, I should have my body back to myself, boobs and all, in two or so years. (Sob, so far away!) I have no plan to extend that timeline with a third child.

I know that may sound harsh, but my husband is old enough that if he wanted three children we'd basically have to have them back to back, and I'm not prepared to do that, physically or mentally. I won't be able to do what my parents did and have a 10-year gap between my sister and me, and my brother. So, I just don't think three is a feasible option. Maybe we could consider adoption for a third, but I don't think my body will be up to the challenge of three kids in quick succession. I just want to feel normal again.

Chapter 24- I Don't Mean to Alarm You, But I Can't See

So the other day I was happily sitting down, munching away on some watermelon and watching an episode of *The Dog Whisperer* when I realized I couldn't see my laptop screen very well. At first I thought I just wasn't concentrating, but when I tried I couldn't focus my eyes properly. It felt a bit like I was cross eyed.

After a puzzling ten minutes I googled pregnancy related vision problems and was presented with information on preeclampsia. For those of you not familiar with it, it isn't good. It's characterized by high blood pressure and protein in the urine, and can lead to eclampsia, a condition that can put mother and baby at risk.

After reading (with difficulty) about it I messaged my husband at his office saying, "I don't mean to alarm you but I can't see properly." I then forwarded him the link to what I'd been reading and asked if I needed to worry. Apparently, he read as far as "can't see" and "low oxygen to the baby" before replying telling me to get my stuff, we were going to the doc immediately.

Of course, by the time he got home my vision had cleared up and I could see again. But we called the doctor, just in case, because according to my husband, "You don't fuck with vision and you don't fuck with oxygen," and they suggested we come in to have my blood pressure checked.

The doctor checked my blood pressure, it was low, and asked a bunch of questions about whether I'd felt I was about to faint when my vision went funny. Now, having fainted a few times before (thank you, anemia) I'm very familiar with what that sensation feels like. It feels like your heart is beating weirdly, your vision goes black around the edges, the blackness slowly closes in, and unless you sit down immediately, everything goes dark. This was different. It was like double vision.

The funniest part was that I hadn't felt very well when we arrived so I'd grabbed a packet of Starburst from the pharmacy and eaten five, just in case my shaky feeling was due to low blood sugar. The doctor asked me what I had eaten recently and when I told her about the five sweets she proceeded to give me a lecture on not eating sugar.

Now, I am the last person she really needed to give that speech to. Those five sweeties were probably the first sweets I'd eaten in months. I almost never eat candy and if the pharmacy had had some fruit, I would have gotten that instead. It's also fairly ironic that a pharmacy in medical center sells candy. I mean, come on! That's like selling cake at a diabetic clinic. It's just stupid.

In the end, the doctor concluded that I had low blood pressure and possibly an ocular migraine (I did have a pretty banging headache over my eye). She told me to take some painkillers with caffeine if it happened again and avoid getting up too quickly (LOL- like I move in any direction quickly at this size).

We left with me apologizing to my husband for being melodramatic. The problem with being a Brit is that we never really say how we actually feel. We just say we're doing fine, regardless of the situation. It's only to our nearest and dearest that we sometimes admit our problems, and even then, we tend to play it down (my grandfather famously said he felt "a bit unwell" right after having a heart attack). But this can become a problem because we never really know when to make a fuss over something or when to just suck it up and deal with it, so we tend not to make a fuss, even when we should.

Thankfully, this was the only unplanned trip to the doctor we've made. Other than that, everything's been progressing as it's supposed to. Even my gestational diabetes test came back fine. Not that I was expecting anything different. I've never showed any symptoms of diabetes, but they scheduled me for a test anyway because apparently, in rare cases, it can present with no symptoms.

The worst part about the diabetes test is that it's a fasting test. Now, I think whoever designed this is suicidal. Why on earth would you schedule a pregnant woman for a test where she can't eat in the morning? Even at this later stage of pregnancy, if I don't eat quickly in the morning I start to feel really sick. It's almost like morning sickness comes back if I don't get some food in me pretty swiftly.

With that in mind, I scheduled the test for 7am. I wanted to get it over so I could have some breakfast ASAP. We rocked up on time only to find they were behind schedule. Okay, firstly, how the hell can you be behind schedule at 7am? Secondly, that's not cool! I had to wait an extra twenty minutes after checking in before I was called for my test and I'll fully admit I was in a bitchy mood when the woman came in to take my blood. I felt super shitty BECAUSE I HADN'T EATEN!

After they took my blood they gave me a sugar bomb. It was a tiny, neon orange bottle of what was supposed to taste like orange soda. I had five minutes to drink it. Even though I was desperate to get some sugar in my system, it took me the whole five minutes to drink it. I don't drink soda of any kind, and even when I used to, I drank the diet versions. I never used to drink full sugar coke because it was just too sweet, but this was even sweeter, by like, a factor of ten. It was pretty gross.

Afterwards, I was led to a waiting room and told they'd draw my blood again in an hour, and then once more an hour after that, but if I threw up from the sugar bomb, the test would have to be stopped and re-done at a later date. Thankfully, the waiting room was opposite the bathroom, just in case, but miraculously I managed to keep it down (though there were a few hairy moments).

The thing that really surprised me was that I had expected my baby to go berserk after all that sugar but she barely moved. Seeing as she tends to bounce around my uterus like a pinball machine whenever I eat melon I had been expecting her to go nuts with the sugar, but she didn't. She just wriggled a bit and then did nothing.

Something that is starting to get on my nerves is that when I'm having my blood taken everyone, and I mean EVERYONE, always chooses the same vein. They've been doing that ever since I started giving blood at age 17. However, I've now had enough needles stuck in the same vein that I'm starting to look a bit like a heroin addict, and at this point, I kind of wish people would stop sticking stuff into me.

I'm sure not all these tests are truly necessary.

Thankfully, when the test was over my husband was waiting with food and I got to cram some bacon in my mouth the moment the clinic door closed. Forget sugar, nothing beats bacon, except perhaps bacon AND avocado.

Chapter 25– Monster Labia and Sexy Time Issues

Okay, we're in the third trimester now and my increased girth is resulting is several problems. Firstly, the most embarrassing: due to the increased pressure on my lower half and increased blood volume, I have monster labia. They literally look so swollen you'd think I'd banged half the army in one go.

Currently, I'm the only one aware of this issue as it's been some time since my husband has taken a close up look down there. I hasten to add this isn't due to a lack of interest on his part, rather due to growing insecurity on mine, not least because it's getting increasingly difficult to do my bikini line. I mean, how do you do something you can't see? I've had to resort to attacking it with the trimmer and just hoping for the best.

My sex drive still hasn't returned but that doesn't mean we don't have sex. We do, probably every 2-3 days. However, despite his assurances that he still finds me "bonerific" and wants to make sure I'm satisfied too, I'm just not really comfortable with him seeing my nether regions in all their throbbing glory. I mean, if it's not already depressing enough that my nipples are practically the same size as my palms, I have to contend with pumped up bits too.

Sex when you're quite far down the line is an awkward thing. Firstly, you have to get a bit creative about which positions you can use. I can't have anyone squash my stomach, so missionary is out. I'm too tired to go on top, so that's out. My arms are already exhausted from heaving myself in and out of chairs, so doggy style is also out. We've ended up choosing a position that's a cross between a right angle and a pair of scissors. Something one of my friends described as "lesbian sex" (not that I'd know but Angelina Jolie, if you're reading, I'd be happy to find out).

Secondly, no one can prepare you for how weird it feels to be kicked while you're having sex. You're supposed to be "in the moment" but you can't be because someone is ramming their foot into your ribcage. Not only is it distracting, it's also off putting. I end up wondering whether my baby's getting annoyed that her dad's wang is banging against her head (because apparently, only she's allowed to collide with my cervix, no one else).

I do feel lucky that my husband still thinks I'm attractive. I did quiz him the other day about whether he'd ever found another pregnant woman attractive. He said not one as heavily pregnant as me, which leads me to think it's possibly an evolutionary thing. It's in his best interests to find the mother of his child attractive as sticking around increases the chances of his offspring's survival.

However, I gather that this isn't always the case. I have read a few blogs and online forums where men have been frank about their feelings towards their pregnant wives' bodies, and some have just found them a massive turn off.

Now, I'm not sure whether they're just referring to things outside a woman's control, such as the size of her boobs and the fact that her stomach simply HAS to expand and get bigger to accommodate a baby, or whether they're referring to an unnecessarily huge weight gain. It's hard to judge, but I'm grateful that despite my growing likeness to a beached whale, my husband still thinks I'm smokin'.

But there is trouble on the horizon. Whilst my husband can easily get his fill at the moment, that won't be the case after I give birth. Not because I'll be too tired, but because apparently, I'll be bleeding for up to 6 weeks as my body heals from the wound created after expelling the placenta (payback for all those missed periods!).

Six weeks may not sound like a long time to some people, but to my husband, that's a lifetime. Normally, he doesn't care about blood and we've been known to have sex while I'm on my period (TMI- sorry). But this will be different. I'll probably be sore and if we have sex too soon there's a risk I could get an infection.

So, the only solutions are: blow jobs or hand jobs. Seeing as I'm not fond of the former when I'm tired (it is a lot of effort), I reckon there'll be a lot of hand jobs going around for the first six weeks of my daughter's life. Who knows, maybe I'll even end up multi-tasking. I can try and breastfeed and give a hand job at the same time. Then when everyone's got what they need from me, I can take a nap.

I know most women will be saying that I shouldn't bother thinking about sex and that my husband should understand, but I reckon one of the reasons we've maintained such a good relationship throughout my pregnancy is due to the fact that sex has never been off the cards, even though I rarely feel "sexy" anymore.

It's hard to feel attractive when you waddle and feel like your back might be broken. Whilst I'm sure my husband gets a good kick out of the back rubs I request. I'm mostly grimacing in pain as he massages the kinks out of my back. And then there's the pelvic pain. Every now and again it feels like I'm being stabbed in the pelvis. Yelping in pain certainly doesn't help "set the mood."

People keep telling me to pamper myself but... how? I struggle to shave my legs at the best of times so I don't think painting my toenails is really on the cards (though my husband has volunteered to do them for me). My idea of pampering at the moment is lying on the sofa with a billion cushions while I watch an entire Netflix series without a shred of guilt.

I'm also getting a bit fed up of people saying "sleep now while you can" because on top of waking up every two hours to pee, I'm now so big that I don't seem to be able to sleep on my back anymore. Meaning I wake up even more because I'm uncomfortable on my side and have to turn over because my hips are hurting.

It's kind of ironic. I've finally found a cure for my restless legs (the midwife was right about the calcium, magnesium and zinc pills helping that) and now I still can't sleep. You'd think your body would have done everything possible to evolve so you'd be in tip top shape to actually deal with a baby when it's born, but noooooo. My body is determined to make the sleep deprivation last as long as physically possible. It's been so long since I slept for more than 3 hours in a row that I don't even remember what it feels like to wake up and think, "I feel great today." And that's likely to last for some years yet. Just thinking about it makes me want a nap.

Chapter 26– Home Birth Changes of Heart

Okay, so I know I previously said I just wanted someone to drug me up to the nines and take the baby out but I've officially found myself having a change of heart. I have definitely decided to do a home birth. My husband has always maintained that it's my decision how to have the baby, but he's secretly pleased, because he wanted to do a home birth in the first place. In his opinion, hospitals are for sick people, and I'm not sick.

It was Ina May's *Guide to Childbirth* that convinced me in the end. I suddenly realized that while hospitals and doctors are great for other medical issues, they seem to have lost the plot somewhat when it comes to childbirth. Maybe it's because nothing is actually wrong with you. Giving birth isn't a medical problem and, for the most part, does not require medical interventions (just a bit of patience, privacy, and time, all of which are in short supply in a hospital).

The idea that someone will induce me because I'm taking too long, or refuse to let me eat or drink, or refuse to let me get up because I have to stay in the position they deem best for birth (which is actually not the best position and only preferred because it's the best position for a forceps delivery), frankly just put me off hospitals. Plus, I don't want to be left in a cold, scary hospital ward, hooked up to a load of wires and tubes. I want to stay with my husband, which I can do at home. Once it's over I'll be able to curl up in bed with him and no one can tell him he has to go home because visiting hours are over.

With the looming deadline of having to pay a hospital deposit for the birth I googled around and found some midwives that do home births. We had our first appointment the other day. First impressions were all good. Firstly, unlike the doctor, she was exactly on time for the appointment. Usually, at the doctors, we would show up and wait up to an hour to be seen. And even then, we'd only be seen by the nurse. We'd still have to wait for the doctor, and when she did finally show up we'd get about ten minutes of her time. All of which was terribly annoying and dull because I had no reception in their office so couldn't even keep myself entertained with silly cat pictures online.

With the midwife, there was no waiting and we got an hour of her time. A WHOLE HOUR. We asked a whole bunch of questions, chatted about random stuff, and at the end of the hour I was set on doing a home birth with her. Out of all the people I'd seen, all the medical professionals, she was the only one who didn't make me feel nervous about what was about to happen. And that meant a lot to me because being nervous about giving birth can make the whole process harder.

The silliest part about switching my birthing plan was telling the doctors that I was going to do a home birth. I was warned that most doctors here in the U.S. totally frown on it and think you're taking stupid risks (blah, blah, blah) and that I should expect a lot of resistance. I put that phone call off for about four days before finally thinking, "Fuck it! It's my body and my decision." Luckily, I didn't have to wrestle the doctor and her objections. I just spoke to the receptionist, told her I was moving and that I'd send a form authorizing the release of my medical records.

Now that we've officially switched to the midwife my anxiety levels about giving birth have reduced significantly. I've done enough research on it that I feel content that my body isn't useless and it will actually be able to do this without drugs and medical interventions, because if we weren't able to have babies without all that paraphernalia we would have died out a long time ago.

One thing a lot of people ask about home births, and a question that we asked, was what the transfer rate was like to hospital. The midwife told us with first time mothers it was about 10%, BUT that the majority of that 10% was women who'd gotten over-excited and run around like a headless chicken and worn themselves out. So, they ended up being transferred because they were tired, wanted the painkillers, and just wanted it to be over with.

I, on the other hand, intend to do no running around whatsoever (like I could at this size). I plan to sit down with a 3,000-piece jigsaw puzzle and maybe a glass of wine (I'm not getting painkillers – let me have that one glass!). Sod running around. I haven't been able to run for months. I don't plan to call everyone I know to excitedly tell them I'm labor either. I'll be pleased to have my daughter out but I can't fake it. I'm just not one of those soppy mums gushing about how desperate they are to have their child in their arms.

I still distinctly remember the first time I saw my brother after he was born. I thought he looked like a pink, runty pig. He sounded like one too, and I was pretty revolted. Newborn babies aren't pretty things. When you say the word "baby" everyone seems to think of a 6 month old, not a wrinkly, gooey blob of fury that is loudly protesting to having been evicted from their cushy life of living inside mum.

Despite my father saying that all babies look like Winston Churchill, I am curious who my daughter will look like. Neither I nor my sister look that much like our parents. We look more like our grandparents on respective sides of the family. So it is possible my daughter won't look like us at all. Furthermore, you can't even be sure of your baby's eye color when they're born. If they're born with blue eyes they could change to brown and you won't know for a couple months what color they'll turn out to be. One of the trippiest things to watch was my brother's eyes changing color. He was born with deep blue eyes, ocean blue, and they gradually changed to brown. For a while they were multi-colored, and it was the weirdest thing to look at, far weirder than people who have one blue eye and one brown.

So, whilst I'm looking forward to my daughter being out, I'm not overjoyed about the fact that I'll have a newborn to deal with. Newborns are, in my opinion, a bit crap. Due to the size of human brains, human babies are born woefully underdeveloped in comparison to other species. Other species can walk, run and deal with their own poop shortly after birth because they're able to gestate to a more reasonable level of development. However, due to our abnormally large heads, we're born underdeveloped because if human babies stayed inside any longer they'd never be able to get out.

The result? A whiny blob that can't walk, communicate beyond crying, see beyond about 18 inches, or hold its head up. Now doesn't that sound fun? And that's not even getting started on the lack of circadian rhythms and ability to hold more than a tablespoon of milk at a time. The more I think about it, the more attractive a puppy sounds.

On the subject of milk, I've actually found myself googling breast pump reviews. I know breast milk is best but I'm not sure I want to do it exclusively. Partially because I know I'll get angry and fed up from feeling like a milking machine, partially because I'd like my husband to be able to do that too so he can bond with our daughter (and I can sleep), partially because so many people frown on breastfeeding in public, and partially because I'd like to share some of the feeding duties.

However, it seems like there are some drawbacks to bottle feeding breast milk. The biggest one as far as I'm concerned is that for some babies once you switch to a bottle you can't go back, and bottle feeding is a lot more hassle. You have to sterilize everything and mess around heating it up and that's a pain to do if you're out or travelling.

The other drawback I'm concerned about is the immunological benefits. Your body actually picks up cues from the baby's saliva about what antibodies it should produce in breastmilk (isn't that neat?), but if you're part bottle feeding, you're a day or two behind what your baby has been exposed to. And if you're exclusively bottle feeding, you're not getting that information at all.

I suppose it all points to the general conclusion that how we evolved to feed our children is the most ideal (if totally annoying and sometimes inconvenient) way to feed them. I intend to try my best to breastfeed but I'm not really enamored by the whole thing like "the breast is best" gang. I have a complicated relationship with my boobs. They were huge as a teenager (we're back to that size now, maybe even bigger) and boys used to tease me about it or point it out. Ever since then I've felt somewhat resentful towards my boobs and pretty emotionally detached from them. In fact, I get no sexual sensation from them at all.

I really don't like people obsessing over my boobs. I hate them when they're huge (like now), and I hate people fussing or playing with them for long. None of this gives me great confidence that I'm going to enjoy having a baby attached to them for a year or more. I guess it's just something I will have to deal with, but if it gets too much then to hell with the naysayers. I'll be switching to a bottle. Until you've walked in my shoes, y'all can suck it.

Chapter 27- Hiccups, Anti-Gravity Tubs, and Magical Poop

At our last visit to the midwife I found out that what had seemed like a weird pulse on my stomach was, in fact, my daughter having a bout of the hiccups. I had never heard anything about babies having hiccups in the womb, but apparently they often do. It can happen when they swallow amniotic fluid. This was news to me, and to my husband, who proceeded to look very confused before finding it all immensely funny as he listened to it.

At the same time, I've also developed hiccups. But not just any hiccups. Singular hiccups. Every now and again I'll just randomly hiccup once, sometimes followed by a burp. I'm not sure whether it's just because my daughter is putting pressure on my diaphragm (that's what hiccups are – a spasm of the diaphragm), but whatever the cause, I get them all the time now. My husband thinks it's cute. I just find it a bit annoying. You're going about your business and suddenly, "Hic!" Talking on the phone when, "Hic!" It doesn't help people take you seriously. I mean, when was the last time you were able to keep a straight face when someone was hiccupping?

At the same appointment we also discussed whether to use a birthing pool. Apparently, being submerged in deep water can do a lot for pain relief, but I already know this because my husband bought me an inflatable hot tub for the back garden. I LOVE IT! It's possibly the best present anyone's ever given me, and because we're in control of the temperature (we set it to body temperature), I can stay in it as long as I want.

Whenever my back starts to hurt too much, or I get bored, or want some sunshine, I just go outside, pull the top off and hop it. It's bliss. Total bliss. Unless you're actually being kicked, pain disappears almost immediately. The first day we got it I went in three times, and I've been in almost every day since it arrived. Best $400 ever spent.

Plus, having your own hot tub does have some additional benefits such as no tan lines. We've set ours up out of the line of sight of any of our neighbors so

I don't have to bother wearing a bikini, because let's face it, at this point there is almost no swimsuit that can contain my boobs. So why even try?

So, with all that in mind, we're going to give the labor tub a whirl. We considered just using the hot tub but it's outside and I don't want to be shrieking down the neighbors while I'm at it. So we decided something indoors would be more practical.

The more I read into what's going to happen during birth the more undignified it becomes. Did you know almost all women poop during labor? Yes? Well I didn't until recently. And frankly, I find that horrifying. I'm the kind of person that gets stage fright at the best of times. In fact, my husband is not allowed in the bathroom if I'm using it. We don't have an open-door policy. So the idea that I'm going to poop in front of him and two other people... UGH!

What's more, guess what happens if I poop in the labor tub? Someone has to fish it out. I'm not sure what's more mortifying, the fact that I'll probably poop or that if I do they'll have to fish it out with a little net thing! (In fact, our birthing kit includes a net and for a while we wondered what they hell it was for.) Can you honestly think of anything more simultaneously hilarious and embarrassing? Of course, everyone tells me I won't care when it happens. And that's true. I probably won't care... when it happens, but what about afterwards?

You know those nights when you just can't sleep so your brain helpfully decides to keep you occupied by reminding you of all the most embarrassing things you've ever done? Well, I'll be able to add "having someone fish my poop out of a tub with a net" to the list. And I'm pretty sure that afterwards, when I'm conscious and not in pain, I'll find that pretty humiliating.

I just don't buy the argument that "it's natural" and "everyone does it." That really doesn't make me feel better about the whole thing. And who exactly is portraying this as natural?! When was the last time you heard an honest depiction about birth? I don't know a single woman who's ever admitted to me that they frequently wet their pants during pregnancy and pooped during birth.

So, if our friends and family don't tell us this stuff, where does our information about birth come from? That's right, the media. Have you ever seen a movie where the onscreen midwife wipes away poop before handing the mum the baby? Of course not! Have you ever read an article from a celebrity admitting they thought birth was shit, literally? Of course not!

Birth is romanticized by almost everyone. They talk about it as if it's a magical experience but I honestly don't remember the last time I was able to describe taking a dump as "magical." My husband, on the other hand... maybe it's a guy thing. Guys are more into their poop than girls. I've never heard a girl say, "It was so big I had to weigh myself afterwards!"

No one ever told me about this crap (pun intended). Or that I'd end up collapsing in pain from my daughter hitting my cervix and the nerves in my back and leg, or that I'd struggle to breathe because my lungs would get so squashed, or that you should never trust a burp because you might just be sick because there's no space for food in your stomach, or that at times I'd struggle to walk due to the pressure on my pelvis. I just feel I'd be a bit less resentful if I'd known a bit more about what I was really in for. Forget all those ads about being miss-sold PPI. I've been mis-sold pregnancy.

Chapter 28- Home Visits, Vagina Swabs, and Placenta Pills

I'm at 36 weeks and officially, as of next week, I'll be able to have a home birth. So, this week our midwife came to see where we live. You know, so she doesn't get lost on the way. We discussed where to put the birthing tub, how we're going to fill it, empty it, and what to cover with plastic sheeting. To be honest, it sounded a bit like it's going to be like a scene from *Dexter*. I got the impression I'll be leaving a trail of blood in my wake. It's a good thing my husband has a strong stomach.

Among the usual urine test (mine almost always resembles water now due to how thirsty I get), I had to do a vagina swab. Of course, if I was still seeing the doctor they probably would have put me in the stirrups, jacked me open and done it. But as my midwife rather bluntly told my husband when he asked, surprised, if I was going to do that swab myself, "She can find her own vagina."

The test was for Group B Strep. This is a standard test in the U.S. but not in the UK. Why might you ask? Because the incidences of babies dying from Group B Strep, even if you have it, are incredibly low. But someone's child probably died from it in the U.S. and the parents sued for negligence and won, and now it's a test everyone has to take. So, up went the cotton bud to be twirled thrice and shoved in the tube for testing.

My midwife does a lot of things differently from the doctors. She wouldn't have made me take the gestational diabetes test unless I'd actually showed symptoms, she doesn't weigh me, and she doesn't poke around inside unless necessary. The only reason she recommended I take this test is in case I have to be transferred to hospital. If you're transferred, unless you have taken the test and know you're negative they'll pump you full of antibiotics on the assumption that your vagina is host to killer bacteria.

Another thing we talked about at the visit was where to deliver the placenta. You see, it doesn't all come out at the same time. The baby comes out first and then, maybe 20 minutes later your placenta will detach and show up. And that's when the bleeding will really start. Great, just what I want after forcing a baby through my nether regions, a river of Satan's wrath.

My midwife says that sometimes mothers like to give birth in the tub and then go over to the bed or sofa to deal with the placenta, perhaps because it's easier to deal with the baby out of the tub. Hospitals treat the baby's arrival in much the same way they treat labor, like a conveyor belt. They want to get the baby out, cleaned, weighed, cord cut and placenta detached as fast as possible. So much so that they sometimes even tug on the umbilical cord to try and detach the placenta from your uterus faster.

If you're not horrified by this, you should be. There's so much wrong with this. Firstly, it's really important for mother and baby to have skin on skin contact for a while. This stimulates all sorts of hormonal things such as breastfeeding, bonding etc. Secondly, cutting the cord too early can cause blood loss to the baby. When you're too hasty to get the whole birthing process done and dusted blood travelling from the baby to the placenta (ya know, to steal your vitamins) can be cut off prematurely, resulting is blood loss for the baby. Not a good thing.

In fact, premature cord clamping (clamping before the blood vessels in the cord stop pulsing) can cause between a 20-50% loss of blood to the baby. That's a lot! It can also cause postpartum hemorrhage, retained placenta, and respiratory distress in the baby. Sounds mad, right? So why the hell are the doctors so bloody hasty about it? Oh, yeah, because time is money <facepalm>.

Once the placenta is out most people just throw it away, but there's a new trend whereby women are ingesting their own placenta. And, as much as I hate to admit it, I'm genuinely considering giving it a try. There's not much scientific evidence on it (published studies) but the theory is it can help with energy levels, boost your milk supply, and help prevent postpartum depression.

I really don't want postpartum depression. I understand there'll be a bit of a hormone come down, but I really don't want the "lying in an abyss of misery" kind of crash. However, having recently watched the first two season of Hannibal on Amazon (I swear I'm a masochist), I really don't think I'll be up to drinking any placenta smoothies. So, I've enquired about having mine dehydrated and turned into pills.

Part of me thinks this is just a new age, hippie thing to do, but then again, if it works, does it matter? Even if it only works as a placebo effect, does it really matter? The woman I contacted (also a midwife) gave me a whole bunch of information on placenta pills, and seeing as it wasn't too expensive, I decided to do it. I'm going for the "better to have it and not need it than need it and not have it" approach. I can always choose not to take them if I change my mind later.

Chapter 29- Impatience, Cervix Banging, and Vaginal Vitamins

Okay, I've reached 38 weeks and I'm officially impatient. I want her out. NOW! I thought things couldn't get much worse, but they have, because she's bigger. Movements that were uncomfortable before are SERIOUSLY painful now. The amount of times I end up poking my own stomach trying to move my daughter off my cervix is just getting ridiculous.

The other day I was happily laying on the sofa, minding my own business, when suddenly, BAM! She attacked my cervix and the nerve in my back at the same time. I was in agony. It was the only time I've seen my husband look genuinely worried. He rushed over and, despite me probably weighing something similar to a baby hippo, he flipped me over onto my other side.

Sometimes changing sides helps the pain. Sometimes it doesn't. Meaning sometimes even when I desperately need a nap, I can't have one, because my f***ing daughter won't let me lie down. She's even disrupting my husband's sleep. Occasionally, he says he wakes up in the night because the mattress is shaking, and it's not me moving. It's my daughter kicking me! Amazingly, as long as she doesn't hit anything that hurts, I manage to sleep through it. But several times I've woken up whimpering.

I just want her to hurry up and come out already. You would not believe the stuff I'm doing in the hope she'll come on time, or even early. I'm having regular sex in the hope that the proglastins in sperm will stop me going past my due date, I'm eating dates because my midwife mentioned she'd read a study that they might help labor be shorter, and I'm putting evening primrose oil up my cooch to try and soften my cervix.

Yes, you read that right. I am putting supplements up my vagina, or more specifically, my husband is. We were recommended this by the midwife to help soften my cervix, which is something that has to happen to get the baby out, and at this point, I'm prepared to try anything (make sure you get the soft gel ones if you intend to try this). However, I can't really reach my bits anymore. I can't get past my stomach very easily. When I try, my daughter's foot usually ends up popping over my ribs and it FREAKING HURTS,

So, like a true man, my husband has taken on the job of shoving a pill up my bits every evening. The first time he took on said duties it was hilarious. A while ago, because my daughter is sitting so low in my pelvis, the midwife suggested he stick a (clean) finger up there sometime and see if he could feel her head. The first opportunity came with the first pill.

The shock on his face was priceless.

"OH, MY GOD! She's RIGHT THERE!"

He couldn't even get his whole finger inside, only about two thirds, and to be honest, I wasn't surprised. My pelvis was so sore that I figured she had to be really low down. But she was basically as low as she could get without actually falling out. He immediately emailed the midwife to tell her about it and she said it was one of the funniest emails she'd ever received.

A day or two later I told my best friend about the evening primrose oil saga and she said, "You've really got to be comfortable with each other for him to do that." I guess we are pretty comfortable. I mean, you have to be to turn to your partner and say, "When you're done brushing your teeth I need you to shove this pill up my vagina." I can't think of any other person I'd be willing to say that to.

My daughter really could come anytime now. So, I've been slowly ticking things off the birth supply list and putting them in one place, doing chores I know I won't care to do once she's born, and doing my best to stay on top of the housework. I've even resorted to doing the ironing to keep myself occupied, and I despise ironing.

People keep telling me I'll get a sudden burst of energy and I'll start "nesting" and want to clean the house from top to bottom and landscape the garden, but that just doesn't seem to be happening. Just like the fabled return of my sex drive in the second trimester… good side effects seem to be skipping me by. I get really tired now. I can only clean one room at a time before I have to sit down and take a break.

Walking is also getting more challenging. I used to frequently waddle to my husband's office and bring him lunch, but even that seems like an insurmountable challenge these days. I know exercise is supposed to be good for a whole host of reasons, but the more I walk the sorer my pelvis becomes. So, at this point I'm somewhat letting the exercise thing slide. There's only so much you can do when you're this spherical.

Even turning over in bed seems like a mammoth task. I sound like a pro tennis player when I attempt to roll over. In fact, turning myself over is now so laborious that I often end up bunching up the sheets as a result, and don't even get me started on getting out of bed. I can't sit up anymore. I have to roll off the bed and just hope I land on my feet.

Recently, I've begun to be plagued in bed by severe urges to roll onto my stomach. I truly detest sleeping on my side. Not least because my stomach is now so big that the sheer weight of it means I can't stay on one side for long without my hips starting to hurt. Meaning I have to turn over, which is in itself another ordeal. It's a vicious cycle which is sometimes totally futile because often when I turn over to give my hip a break my daughter decides she doesn't like the way I'm facing and thus starts to kick me and squirm her head on my cervix to make her feelings known.

Basically, what it all adds up to is me wanting laugh like a crazy woman whenever someone says to me "sleep now while you can." Sleep now? Are you freaking MAD? I haven't slept properly for almost a year! I ache in places no one should ache and there's a wriggling alien inside me making my life hell. At this point I'll be glad to get on to regular sleep interruptions like feeding and diaper changing. It beats being woken up feeling like you're being stabbed in the vagina any day.

Chapter 30– Looming Due Dates, Google Paranoia, and Breastfeeding Issues

Like for most pregnant women my due date has been looming in my mind like some terrible exam. I find myself lying in bed, reading on my phone, essentially cramming revision on what I'm supposed to do when it happens, what the signs of labor are, what I need to have to hand, breastfeeding tips, you name it. It's a far cry from when I spent my internet time scrolling through cat memes and shoes I couldn't afford.

Now that I'm only a few days away from my due date we've put plastic sheeting on the bed under the mattress cover, in case my water breaks in the middle of the night, and I'm on high alert for any symptom of anything happening. I repeat: we are at battle stations!

Signs of labor include a bloody show (blood in your underpants), loss of your mucus plug (in case you didn't know, while you're pregnant your cervix becomes clogged with mucus to protect against infection), your waters breaking (this could either be a trickle or a gush), and contractions.

However, I've had no sign of anything. Nada. Niente. Zip. Lots of women online ask questions about how to tell the difference between Braxton hicks contractions (fake labor) and true labor, but as far as I can tell I've not even had fake contractions. My body has literally shown no interest whatsoever in indicating when this show might get on the road.

The closer I get to my due date the more I start wondering if everything is a sign of labor. The internet is a double-edged sword. It's great to have so much information and advice at your fingertips, but sometimes it can just make you paranoid. You end up googling "headaches and labor", "nausea and labor", "loose stools and labor", "feeling weird and labor", "when will I fucking go into labor?!"

People keep contacting me too, asking how I'm doing and giving me all sorts of stupid advice. You wouldn't believe the old wives tales that pervade about how to bring labor on. So far I've been told to: eat pineapple, bounce on a ball, go for long walks (does to the fridge and back count?), have sex, drink balsamic vinegar, and eat curry. The only one on that list that might actually do anything is the sex.

The reason sex might actually help is because in order to give birth your cervix needs to soften and thin out and sperm contains proglastins, hormones that actually help that happen. However, I've been having pretty regular sex since day one. I don't think we've ever gone more than 4 days without it but I'm not seeing anything as a result.

In reality, the only thing that's going to start labor is the baby. When the baby is ready they'll send hormones out that start the whole process going. It's just that as modern women, we're not used to having to be patient and wait around for someone else's unknown schedule. Today's women are used to being in control, having known deadlines and meeting them. Perhaps that's why we all go so loopy and are so eager to induce when things don't go to our plan.

Quite a lot of people are checking in with me at this point. Asking how I'm doing and stuff, but really, there's not much to report. Yes, I'm still pregnant. No, there's no signs of that changing. Yes, I'm fed up. No, I won't miss being pregnant. No, I'm not scared because... did I mention I was fed up?

I'm also getting a lot of strangers asking me when I'm due. Apparently, now mere days away from being due, it's obvious enough that I'm pregnant, and not fat, for strangers to ask me when I'm due. I've got to admit, as much as I want my daughter out, I'm trying not to place too much significance on the due date. After all, it's not an exact science.

Due dates are calculated by either your last period, or an ultrasound (or both). But they're not set in stone, because what you really need to know to calculate a more accurate date is when in your cycle you ovulate. Not all women ovulate at the 14-day mark. So, if you ovulate later in your cycle, your due date (as calculated by your period) can be off by up to a week or more.

In fact, in France they don't consider you overdue until after 41 weeks, which, according to my midwife, is very sensible, seeing as most first time mothers are, on average, eight days late. So all this obsession over the 40 week mark got me to thinking, what problems does taking babies out before they're ready cause?

One of the things I've been looking into recently is why so many women online complain about breastfeeding being hard. I know it won't be a walk in the park as far as my nipples are concerned but the amount of problems people seem to have in just getting their baby to feed seemed a little odd to me. I mean, what do indigenous people do without lactation consultants? Surely babies that don't nurse would otherwise die? And judging by how many babies seem to have problems surely we'd have died out as a species by now.

On a hunch, I did a little research into whether inducing labor before the baby is really ready to come out has any impact on breastfeeding. I came across a good article about the benefits of waiting and how your baby is developing right up until they come out, but what really caught my attention wasn't the content of the article. It was a comment from a lactation consultant underneath the article.

She commented saying that over the years she had observed so many babies that had been induced that had feeding problems. Her theory was that the babies sucking reflexes weren't properly developed because the baby had been forcibly ejected before it was ready.

Now, whilst this is just information from one person somewhere on the internet, it does kind of make sense when you think about it. Due to impatience, we're cutting babies time short in the womb, so it's hardly surprising they're not performing the way we want them to once they're out. I'm pretty sure if you unexpectedly cut my revision time for an exam I'd perform badly too. As tough as it is, and bar any true medical emergencies, it's probably best to let babies decide when they want to come out. Ya know, like nature intended.

Chapter 31- Pregnant Forever

Yes, my due date has come and gone and here I am, five days overdue. I had prepared myself for this, so I wasn't too upset when my due date came and went. But the more days that tick by the more annoyed I'm getting by the kicks and squirming. Unfortunately, when you feel like you're being stabbed in the vagina and have shooting pain down your back and inner thigh you lose affection pretty darn quickly for your baby. I have recently been known to poke my stomach and shout, "Cut out the crap! If you want space to move you have to come out!"

I sent my sister a ranty email to that effect and her reply was classic:

Re. your poor vagina, maybe she's kind of testing the door? ('Like is it this way? Like, am I supposed to come out here? Like, is this the exit right here? Cos I swear people are talking on the other side...how does it open? I also swear it's getting smaller in here, and I'm kind of bored, so do feel like coming out... maybe... am I supposed to come out right here?')

I'd say talk to your vagina and maybe even wave a toy in front of it to coerce her to come out of it. Phrases such as 'here, girl' and patting the area right in front of your vagina might also help, along with mentioning all the cool kids shows she's missing by staying in there.

If you're feeling like you're losing affection for her because she's a little person beating you up from the inside, that's understandable. It sounds a bit like being possessed. I dunno...I think it takes a ridiculously happy (and possibly even masochistic) sucker to "enjoy" this leg of it, but keep an eye on how you're feeling once she's out.

I feel for you.

I feel for me too. I'm totally okay with wallowing in my own pity party right now. You're essentially in limbo after you reach 40 weeks. Chances are you've already done all the baby related tasks such as setting up a nursery, cooking and freezing extra food, and cleaning all the things you know you won't be doing after the baby's born. So, there's not much to distract yourself with.

There's also nothing left to indicate baby progress. We're at the end of the "what size is my baby in relation to a fruit?" chart (she's now the size of a watermelon, in case you wanted to know). There's no new information on what your baby is doing development-wise (other than getting fatter), so it's easy to find yourself asking, "What the fuck are they doing in there? Just hanging out and torturing me for their own amusement?"

The most annoying thing about being overdue is people asking you if you're still pregnant. It's like, well, yeah. OBVIOUSLY! There ought to be some sort of rule whereby unless notified otherwise, everyone just assumes you're pregnant. I mean, I'll tell you when there's a baby. You don't have to ask. You'll either be receiving nauseating baby pictures or one of me glugging a big glass of wine.

I almost feel like I've reached a resigned point where I've just accepted that I'll be pregnant forever and this baby is never coming. In my mind I know she can't stay in there forever, but SO much time has gone by that struggling to get out of chairs, not being able to find a single comfy position to sleep in, and backaches have just become the norm. I don't even remember what it felt like to be able to swing my legs out of bed in the morning and walk to the bathroom without having to grab onto something for support.

I've been trying to keep myself occupied and have taken to doing tasks I'd totally ignore otherwise, such as de-greasing the oven fan and de-limescaling the dishwasher. You may want to call this nesting behavior, but I don't think it is. I'd made a point of being on top of things in the run up to my due date that there's just not much left to distract me other than these tasks. I've even started eyeing up the garage and the garden as potential distraction projects.

I saw my midwife again yesterday and, as usual, everything looks great. We talked a bit about what we'd do if I was still pregnant in a week's time because there are some natural things you can try to bring on labor that aren't just old wives tales. One possibility is acupuncture, sweeping the membranes, and as a last resort I can try castor oil.

Sweeping the membranes is where the midwife has a rummage inside and gently separates the bag of waters from the cervix in the hope of stimulating proglastins (one of the labor hormones). Apart from this being an uncomfortable experience, there is a small chance that if your practitioner isn't careful they could accidentally break your waters. So really, the simplest way of getting proglastins "up there" is probably still sex (sorry, I know some of you won't want to hear that).

The theory with castor oil is that stimulating your bowels to empty may trigger labor because for the most part, women do tend to have a bit of a "clear out" before they go into labor. I was warned that if I seemed to be pooping lots it could be a sign I'd soon go into labor. And whilst not as effective as drugs, castor oil is much safer as a method of inducement. In one study it brought on labor in almost 9% of 11,000 women, which is more than can be said for eating curry. (As a side note, bearing in mind you'll probably poop during labor, I'd question eating that curry if I were you.)

At my appointment, the midwife asked if I wanted to get checked to see if anything was happening down there but we decided not to bother. I see so many women online complaining that they're overdue and only so many centimeters dilated, or so many percent effaced. What they don't seem to realize is that it really doesn't matter how dilated and effaced you are. It has absolutely no bearing whatsoever on when you'll go into labor. You could be 3cm dilated for weeks before anything happens and you could be 0cm and go into labor that evening. Much like weighing yourself, bringing math into the equation (pardon the pun) isn't helping anything right now. It just gives you one more thing to obsess over.

One of the things that has surprised me is that as annoying as being overdue is, I have the feeling that other people are getting more annoyed for me than I am for myself. I am really uncomfortable. I don't sleep well. I seem to have to hold my stomach up with my hands to be able to empty my bladder properly. The pressure on my pelvis is worse than ever but still, it seems to be my friends and family that are getting the most wound up over it.

Maybe I've just given up caring. Like when you know you're going to fail a test and you just accept it and let it happen. Everyone else is stressing about "when the baby's going to come" and I'm just sitting in the hot tub in the garden going, "Ooh! Look! A butterfly."

Chapter- 32 Labor, Assplosions, and Diva Babies

The other day I saw one of our neighbors in the drive and she asked me if I've had any contractions. I told her I couldn't tell because I wasn't sure what I was looking for. She just said "You'll know." And funnily enough, she was right.

So, there I was, 8 days late, minding my own business, when it began to feel a bit like my stomach was getting tense and then relaxing. However, seeing as I couldn't tell the difference between the "tightening" people described as early labor and my baby simply moving, I decided to pay no attention to it, and sat down with my 3,000-piece jigsaw.

An hour or two later my husband came home and asked if we needed to go to the store (because I'd eaten all the fruit… again). I agreed and rushed to use the bathroom before we went but when I went to wipe there was something red on the tissue. For a moment, I sat there confused. Was that blood? I hadn't seen that for a while. So, I wiped again just to be sure, and yep. It was blood.

My "bloody show" (in my head it always sounds like I'm swearing in John Cleese's voice when I say that phrase) had materialized. It was my first recognizable sign of real labor. I texted my midwife to let her know and after confirming the weird tightening I was having was contractions she advised me to get an early night as it could be a long haul. I promised I would, but first we were going to the store. After all, I was out of melon, and this simply would not do.

As we walked around the store it became evident that my contractions were getting stronger so I stubbornly insisted on pushing the trolley, mostly so I had something to hold onto. To my husband's credit, he took the news that a train had started that couldn't be stopped pretty well, and was only mildly over-protective about me not carrying anything.

When we got home we decided to try and time the contractions because they seemed to be pretty close. We were expecting a long pre-labor because that's what everyone had told us was normal for first time mothers, but these were every four to five minutes. So, we decided not to wait and to set up everything we were supposed to while keeping an eye out for the active labor phase.

Active labor is defined as contractions that last for one minute and are three minutes apart from each other for at least an hour. When you reach that stage you call the midwife (or go to the hospital). Seeing as I was banned from any helping with any serious tasks I left my husband to blow up the birthing tub and cover everything in plastic and retreated to the bathroom.

I can only describe what happened next as an "assplosion." I spent the next who knows how long sitting on the loo expelling everything inside me in between contractions that were now serious enough to cause me to yelp and grip onto the shower door handle for support. I must have passed about 7 stools and at one point I even recognized some lettuce I'd eaten at lunch. It was the mother of all poop sessions and had I been a man I would have bragged about it to my mates.

Afterwards I did my best to go to sleep but I really couldn't. The pain was too distracting and far too frequent. After moaning into my pillow and crushing my husband's hand I gave up on the prospect of sleep and got up. For some reason the contractions seemed to hurt more when I was lying down. So, I went to stand by the bathroom sink.

At about 11pm on yet another bathroom trip there was a weird pop and a small gush. My waters had broken. I texted my midwife and she called to check up on me. In between pain rushes I managed to confirm that I'd like her to come over now. I wasn't sure if it was too early, but I wanted her there.

She arrived no more than twenty minutes later (the second midwife shortly thereafter) to find me standing stark naked in front of the sink, having soaked two towels with various fluids (blood, amniotic fluid, some mucus gunk), gripping the countertop as if my life depended on it as the contractions continued to get stronger. Then she did something amazing. She pushed on either side of my hips with her hands and the pain suddenly got better. I could have cried. It was like she had magic hands.

She quickly checked on my progress (I was fully dilated – we were going at full pelt) and coached us through a few contractions, telling me to sink into a squat and make low noises (I tried, but I felt pretty silly), before disappearing to get set up with everything. I put my husband in charge of hip pressing, and we labored on. But there was a problem. The labor tub was filling with water that was too hot and it was taking ages to cool it down. In the meantime, the midwife suggested we hop in the shower. So, we did.

Luckily, on a random trip to Home Depot my husband had seen a suction handle you could attach to the shower wall and thought it was so cool he'd bought it. Sometimes I tell him off for impulsive purchases, but this time I was glad he had bought that, because I was clinging onto it and the soap dish for dear life as my legs shook from the effort of what can only be described as the world's most intense squat workout.

Then something changed. I stopped yelling and made a grunt. I was pushing and it was not a conscious decision. They're right when they say you don't need to be told when to push and you certainly don't need someone shouting at you like some over-muscled personal trainer. The midwife appeared, having heard the change in tone, and, with some padding bunched between my legs, we made a rush down the stairs before another contraction could start.

I hopped in the birthing tub, shortly followed by my husband, who had been walking around all this time in a pair of speedos, and gripped the handle. Then the show really started moving. My husband was still on hip squashing duty so I ended up gripping the hands of both the midwives in turns as they did stuff (no idea what). At this point I wasn't capable of making low noises. I was being unabashedly loud with the pushes.

It seemed to last forever but I'm told that it was actually only 45 minutes of pushing before I was instructed to quickly get out of the tub. The midwife had seen something in the mirror she'd been using to check my progress, but I wasn't about to ask what. I just did as I was told and got out of the damn tub.

The next part I'm rather fuzzy on. I am told that my daughter had her hand up by her face like a true damsel in distress, which was acting like a break, slowing things down. That's why I had to get out of the tub, so the midwife could move her hand out of the way. I remember being told to give some extra oomph to my pushes and I remember grabbing the other midwife. And then the pain ended. She was out.

Chapter 33– The Afterbirth

The relief you feel when you finally push a baby out is somewhat indescribable. The baby was out, but I wasn't paying any attention to the wet little bundle being passed between my legs. I was having what they call "a natural pause" which I would describe as "catching my breath after one helluva workout."

My daughter was placed in my arms and I was helped/rushed over to the couch (which was also covered in plastic), and we were both covered in blankets. Once we were settled and warm, I finally got a chance to look at the person I'd been carrying around for 41 weeks and one day. She looked much as I had expected her to: covered in goop. In fact, the midwives were surprised at how much vernix (a white waxy substance) was covering her skin. Most babies that are "overdue" don't have much left, but my daughter was liberally coated in the stuff. In the hospital they rub the vernix into the baby's skin, but my midwives didn't. They just left her alone and in absorbed into her skin itself. No intervention necessary.

Next came what they refer to as "the afterbirth." You've pushed out the baby but you still have to push out its support system: the placenta. Luckily, because the placenta has no bones it's a fairly pain free experience, and like they say, the way has already been paved, so it wasn't hard to do. The midwife waited until the blood in the cord had stopped pulsing, gave it a very gentle test tug to see if the placenta had detached, and told me to push.

Out came a big squishy blob about the size of my liver. I was actually surprised at how big it was, and that it, my daughter, and all that water had managed to fit in my stomach. It's like my uterus had turned into the TARDIS and the fact that I hadn't gotten any stretch marks seemed even more remarkable.

The placenta was plopped into a freezer bag and placed next to me. While all this had been going on, my daughter had rooted around on my chest until she'd found my boobs, latched on fiercely, and was refusing to let go, so we decided to wait until she was done before cutting the cord and doing the newborn exam.

In the meantime, it was time to inspect the damage. Because my daughter had had her hand up it had made things a little tight on space, and somewhat inevitably, I had torn down there. To be perfectly honest, I hadn't felt it, and I still couldn't feel it (there must have been some pretty epic levels of endorphins in my system).

It wasn't a deep tear but it was a long one. The midwife cleaned me up and numbed the area before deciding to call in backup for the stitches as mine were, apparently, going to be tricky ones. As we waited for another midwife nearby to stop over and sew me up my husband suddenly remembered he'd bought about six bars of chocolate for the birth and hadn't had a chance to eat any of it. Everything had happened too fast.

We broke out the chocolate and, as the midwife cleaned up the meconium my daughter had pooped all over my stomach to do the newborn exam (again, I didn't notice or care – what was one more bodily fluid at this point?), we began placing bets on how much she weighed. Guesses were in the 7-8 pound range. We were all wrong. She weighed 9 pounds. Everyone was surprised because she wasn't very pudgy, except for me. I knew she was heavy. I'd felt every pound of that on my cervix. It turned out she was just long, rather than fat, which made sense seeing as her head had been about two inches from the world and her feet had still been jammed in my ribs.

When I had my wits about me enough I decided to ask if I'd pooped during the birth. Apparently, all that had come out was about two pea sized blobs which had sunk to the bottom of the birthing tub. My earlier assplosion had done a good job of clearing the pipes, and I was pretty grateful for it. Despite my lack of modesty (I'd forgone a bra and just decided to be naked during the whole event), I don't think my pride could have taken watching someone chase a big floater around the birthing tub with a net.

Newborn exam over, my husband cut the umbilical cord, severing my daughter's connection to the placenta in the Ziploc bag, and got his first chance to hold her. To his credit, he didn't cry. He did very well throughout the whole thing. There was only one part where he almost cried and that was when I got out of the tub for the final pushes. I had been fairly oblivious to most things at that point but I had (briefly) noticed he'd looked upset.

Women go on and on about how nothing men go through compares to the pain of labor but no one ever seems to mention how painful it is to watch someone you love be in serious pain and be powerless to help them. I think men deserve a little credit for that. It can't be easy. It may not be physical pain, but it's certainly mental pain.

Finally, the midwife who was going to stitch me up appeared and donned the kind of head torch people wear to go cave diving. Now, I know my bits were probably stretched beyond all conceivable belief, but I wouldn't have gone as far as to describe them as "a cave."

Nevertheless, I was numbed up again, just for good measure, and stitched up. The last task required of me was to use the bathroom and get into bed. With a little help, I waddled with a towel between my legs to the bathroom and the moment my butt hit the seat my bladder admitted defeat and without even a shred of stage fright, I peed (yes, all dignity was gone). The midwife squirted an herbal peri wash to help with any stinging but I was numb from the stitches, so I felt no pain (thankfully). Finally, it was time to go up the stairs to bed.

Never in my life have I found it such hard work to climb stairs. Everything ached, my back, my legs, my ribs… even my throat and voice hurt from all the yelling. I gripped both the banister and the midwife and, gasping for breath, we made it up the stairs. Though, I confess, I had to stop halfway up to take a rest. I'm not sure any walk has ever been harder, except perhaps my first steps as a baby, but I don't remember those, so they don't count.

Finally, at about 5:30am, settled in bed with my daughter on my chest and my husband by my side, after assuring me I'd be checked on the following day, the midwives left. It was now just the three of us, snuggled up for some sleep. It was just how I'd wanted it to be: us three, at home in our own bed, safe and warm and not a hospital gown in sight.

Chapter 32– The Postpartum Period

Once the euphoria (or drugs) from birth wear off you suddenly realize that you're responsible for the tiny bundle in your lap. This little person is now wholly dependent on you. Even for the most capable of us, it's a daunting task. We're so used to putting our own needs first these days that the prospect of simply not being able to take a shower whenever we want to is enough to make us baulk and run the other direction.

I'm not going to go into great detail about this part of pregnancy because once your baby is born there are so many books, resources, and people to tell you what to do, and each parent has to find their own parenting style. What I will say is that there are two key virtues you need when looking after a newborn: flexibility and patience. All those things you thought you'd never do, you'll do them. Whatever schedules you thought you'd keep, that'll go out of the window. And you'll waste more time than you ever thought just checking your child is still breathing.

During pregnancy I had determinedly said I would never sleep with my baby in the bed for fear of crushing her. But guess what? Once she was there I didn't even bother trying to get her to sleep in the basinet that I'd kept by my bed for a month "to get used to." She spent her first day sleeping either on me or next to me and when it came to bedtime I ended up texting my midwife to ask if it was safe for her to sleep with me. She assured me my mothering instincts would make sure I didn't sleep deeply and that it would be okay. And she was right.

My daughter has slept in the bed with us since then. Sometimes she sleeps by my side but when she's being fussy I hold her on my chest and cocoon myself with the body pillow so it's impossible for me to roll over. It does mean that I get less snuggle time with my husband, but it also means we all get more sleep, which at this point, is probably more important. Lack of sleep leads to frayed tempers and frayed tempers aren't good with small children.

The other thing you have to bear in mind is that babies don't cry just to piss you off. They mostly cry because something is wrong or because stuff is scary. Everything is new to them, so it's not unreasonable that they should be clingy and alarmed by almost everything. My daughter cries when she's hungry, needs changing, doesn't like being changed, has the hiccups, has gas, is being bathed, doesn't want to be put down... The list goes on, but she rarely cries for no reason.

As loud and grating as baby cries can be, you just have to try to stay calm and trust yourself. You will figure out what's wrong. You just need time to learn how to interpret the cries, and respond accordingly. I actually had to point out to my husband that mimicking our daughter crying wasn't actually helping anything and that he should try "shushing" noises instead. It's a bit like when dogs bark. If you bark back they don't stop barking. They think you're joining in and bark more.

And finally, you have to be patient with yourself. It takes time to heal from such a huge event and you need to be prepared to do very little for longer than you want to, especially if you have stitches. I didn't leave the house beyond the end of the driveway for two weeks. In fact, I didn't leave the bedroom but to go to the bathroom for three days, and even then I walked like John Wayne the whole way.

Life does get easier but those first few weeks until you're healed up enough to feel semi-normal will seem unendingly long. I can't tell you how many Amazon Prime and Netflix series I went through in the first few weeks. It must have been over fifteen. And I can't tell you how annoyed I got at my boobs leaking (yes, you can buy breast pads but I hate sleeping in a bra), and my stitches making each bathroom trip a traumatic, stinging ordeal (top tip: lean as far forward as you can, use a cup or buy a Shewee to catch your pee so it doesn't touch any sore bits, and invest in an antiseptic numbing spray such as Dermoplast). But as with all things, the annoyances come to pass.

Looking down at my daughter now I am reminded of what everyone kept saying to me during pregnancy: "It'll all be worth it in the end." I suppose they're right. She is worth it. But you'll never catch me saying that to a pregnant woman. Pregnant women don't want to hear that. They just want someone to agree and say, "Yes. Pregnancy is fucking shit. Period."

About the Author

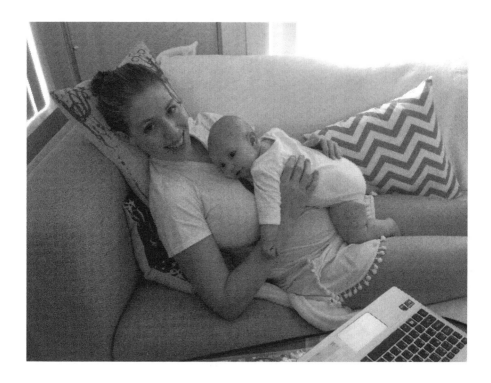

Jocelyn Hayes is a British writer living in California with her high-maintenance daughter and Canadian husband. She is a baking addict, coffee snob, and lover of all things sparkly.

View other Black Rose Writing titles at www.blackrosewriting.com/books and use promo code **PRINT** to receive a **20% discount** when purchasing.

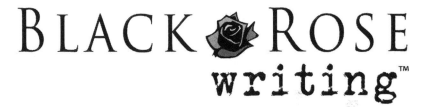

Printed in Great Britain
by Amazon